Behavioral Objectives— Evaluation in Nursing

BEHAVIORAL OBJECTIVES— EVALUATION IN NURSING

Second Edition

DOROTHY E. REILLY
R.N., Ed.D., F.A.A.N.

Professor of Nursing
College of Nursing
Wayne State University
Detroit, Michigan

APPLETON-CENTURY-CROFTS/New York

80 81 82 83 84 / 10 9 8 7 6 5 4 3 2 1

Prentice-Hall International, Inc., London
Prentice-Hall of Australia, Pty. Ltd., Sydney
Prentice-Hall of India Private Limited, New Delhi
Prentice-Hall of Japan, Inc., Tokyo
Prentice-Hall of Southeast Asia (Pte.) Ltd., Singapore
Whitehall Books Ltd., Wellington, New Zealand

Library of Congress Cataloging in Publication Data

Reilly, Dorothy E
  Behavioral objectives—evaluation in nursing.

  First ed. (1975) published under title:
Behavioral objectives in nursing, evaluation of
learner attainment.
  Includes bibliographical references and index.
  1. Nursing—Study and teaching.   2. Lesson
planning.   I. title.
RT71.R48   1980   610.73′07′11   80-10386
ISBN 0-8385-0634-8

Text Design: Ann Gold

PRINTED IN THE UNITED STATES OF AMERICA

To My Students

Contents

Preface

The decision to write a new edition of a book is not taken lightly by the author, for such an endeavor must be supported by the need for new content addressed to increasing knowledge in the area or including new areas that will enrich the book and facilitate its use by the consumer.

This edition incorporates both aspects; some areas are updated while some content is new to the book. The changes reflect feedback from students and colleagues who use the book as well as the author's own experiences in both using the book and conducting workshops and conferences throughout the United States and Canada.

The basic premise of the book remains as stated in the preface of the first edition: "This book deals with the WHAT and the HOW of evaluation with focus on the relationship between these two variables and emphasizes the need for nurse teachers to develop greater creativity and flexibility in their evaluation of the predetermined behavioral objectives." Reviews and comments from users have supported the content of the book and the format by which the content was developed.

One change, however, seemed necessary—that is the change in title. Because the title of the first edition was so lengthy, the book often was referred to as the "one on behavioral objectives," thus negating the true nature of the book, which was to show the relationship between behavioral objectives and evaluation as well as to acknowledge the content relevant to the evaluative process and its strategies. The title selected for the second edition seeks to address this concern.

Major revision of content occurs in four areas of the book: the theory of nursing in Chapter 2; the affective domain in Chapter 4; the principles for preparing multiple recognition items in Chapter 7; and concepts of clinical practice evaluation in Chapter 10. Chapter 4 also includes a list of behavioral terms appropriate for use in writing objectives for all levels of the three taxonomies.

Two new chapters have been incorporated, and Chapter 5 has been augmented by a more specific discussion of hte leveling process. Suggestions for program objectives are offered and the process of leveling is presented either by use of the taxonomies or by increasing the complexity of variables with which behaviors are related.

The new Chapter 6 is the result of a need arising from the increased use of continuing education as an update process for practicing nurses. Since the objectives stated for a program are in essence a contract with the consumer, more care needs to be taken to assure that the objectives are relevant and capable of being evaluated.

Chapter 9, which also was added to this edition, resulted from numerous requests by users of the first book. The focus of the chapter is on the process of test construction. primarily criterion-referenced testing, and illustrates the process for identifying the critical elements or test units within any behavioral objective.

The author is most indebted to students and colleagues who have used the first edition of the book and so generously offered comments and suggestions. It is the hope that this new edition will be even more helpful to individuals participating in the development of and the teaching in educational programs within nursing or other health fields.

DOROTHY E. REILLY

Preface to the First Edition

This book is designed for nursing teachers and for prospective nursing teachers. It aims to help them increase the nursing teacher's competency in the difficult task of evaluating learning achievement, and it maintains that this evaluation process can best be accomplished through the use of behavioral objectives. It is the author's hope that it will prove useful for schools of nursing, for staff development programs whether in hospitals or other health agencies, for continuing education, and for community health education.

The evaluation component of education often can evoke feelings of insecurity, inadequacy, and guilt on the part of nurse educators, especially as they address themselves to the clinical practice portion of the program. Many of these feelings may result from the greater emphasis placed on the HOW of evaluation (procedures to be used) rather than on the WHAT of evaluation (object). Accentuation of methodology over substance has often led to some incongruency between the two, so that evaluation results are invalid in terms of the original intent. Furthermore, failure to identify clearly the object of evaluation has often led to the practice of limiting tests to the evaluation of the cognitive skill of remembering information. Also questionable is the tendency to limit clinical evaluation to skills in technical procedures and to compliance to the behavioral norms of the practice setting.

The current trend toward the use of behavioral objectives as a basis for program development and evaluation has much potential for facilitating the teaching-learning process through the identification of the WHAT.

This book deals with the WHAT and the HOW of evaluation with focus on the relationship between these two variables and emphasizes the need for nurse teachers to develop greater creativity and flexibility in their evaluation of the predetermined behavioral objectives.

The WHAT of evaluation is presented as a discussion of behavioral objectives in nursing in relation to the

1. Derivation to provide for relevancy of these objectives.
2. Development of behavioral objectives. Many books are available for explaining the technique of objective writing; this aspect will receive limited attention.
3. Use of behavioral objectives in a nursing program.
4. Application of the taxonomy of learning behaviors to nursing behaviors.

The HOW of evaluation is presented as a discussion in relation to the

1. Concept of evaluation as derived from one's perspective on the process.
2. Identification of evaluative approaches appropriate to nursing programs.

The two variables—WHAT and HOW— are brought together through the demonstration of

1. Application of each evaluative approach to a specific behavior or to several behaviors.
2. Multi-evaluative approaches for any given specific behavior.

This book is offered in response to requests from my students and from nursing colleagues throughout the country with whom I have shared my ideas and thinking in consultations, institutes, workshops, and other professional forums. These students and colleagues have encouraged me in developing my approach, have challenged me to refine my thinking, and have contributed to my own growth. Indeed, they have been true critics.

Acknowledgment is extended to Margaret Shetland, former Dean at the College of Nursing, Wayne State University, for supporting my endeavors and to those colleagues in the College of Nursing who provided that special type of caring which made the writing of this book a pleasurable and worthwhile experience.

In an endeavor such as writing, the author is enriched by being assisted by individuals who give not only of their expertise, but also of themselves. As this book reaches its final stage of development, I am especially indebted to four such individuals. A special recognition is extended to my dear friend, Hope Brophy, who cast her journalistic eye over the manuscript to insure that it met high editorial standards.

Three individuals, Maria Phaneuf, professor emeritus of public health nursing at the College of Nursing, Wayne State University, LaVaughn Sharp, director of the Grace Hospital School of Nursing in Detroit, and Margretta Styles, Dean of the College of Nursing, Wayne State University, gave unstintingly of their time, humanness, and expertise as readers of the original manuscript. Their thoughtful assessment and constructive criticisms contributed to the refinement of the manuscript.

My deepest appreciation is extended to my mother and to everyone who in his/her own way showed faith in my efforts and provided me with the support necessary for realizing my own dream, the publication of this book.

DOROTHY E. REILLY

Behavioral Objectives— Evaluation in Nursing

1 Instructional Accountability

A CURRICULUM FABLE

One time the animals had a school. The curriculum consisted of running, climbing, flying, and swimming, and all the animals took all the subjects.

The Duck was good in swimming, better, in fact, than his instructor, and he made passing grades in flying, but he was practically hopeless in running. Because he was low in this subject, he was made to stay in after school and drop his swimming class in order to practice running. He kept this up until he was only average in swimming. But average is acceptable, so nobody worried about that except the Duck.

The Eagle was considered a problem pupil and was disciplined severely. He beat all the others to the top of the tree in the climbing class, but he used his own way in getting there.

The Rabbit started out at the top of the class in running, but he had a nervous breakdown and had to drop out of school on account of so much make-up work in swimming.

The Squirrel led the climbing class, but his flying teacher made him start his flying lessons from the ground instead of the top of the tree down, and he developed charleyhorses from overexertion at the take-off and began getting C's in climbing, D's in running.

The practical Prairie Dogs apprenticed their offspring to a Badger when the school authorities refused to add digging to the curriculum.

At the end of the year, an abnormal Eel that could swim well, run, climb, and fly a little was made valedictorian.

(Author unknown)

The highest honors in this school went to an abnormal eel!! Are the learners who come out of our programs abnormal eels, i.e., abnormal men and women as nurses? What goals direct our programs, what do we evaluate, and what criteria do we use for this evaluation? Can we meet the criterion of accountability for our educational programs?

ACCOUNTABILITY IN EDUCATIONAL ENDEAVORS

Evaluation is a term well known to educators and students in the American society, although its interpretation and impact vary widely among groups and among individuals. Accountability is a term currently used by educators and employed in a sense consistent with its use by many other groups in modern society.

Are the terms *evaluation* and *accountability* synonymous as some references seem to suggest? Both terms connote a process concerned with determining the quality of a substance, action, or event. *Accountability*, however, implies an additional dimension, that of being answerable for quality.

Nursing, along with other professional groups and institutions serving our society, is increasingly held accountable for the quality of service it provides. This entails assessment of goals, resources, actions, and products in light of society's needs and resources.

As nursing teachers in whatever setting we practice, we too will be held more and more accountable for our actions. We must answer to the student, to society, to our profession, to the institution offering the program, and to ourselves.

Society has accepted and legitimized nursing as an institution important to its health care. Is society receiving the nursing care it needs, or is it getting the nursing care we *think* it needs or deserves? Where is the consumer of our services fitting into deliberations on the kind of nursing for which we are preparing practitioners? As educators, we must respond to society's concern about the rising cost of preparing nurses. Can we demonstrate that the nurses sent into the health care system have made a difference for the better in the quality of health care provided in proportion to the scope of their educational preparation?

The rapidity of change within all subsystems of our society challenges nursing to make its own changes so that its participation in the health delivery system is compatible with society's needs and nursing's areas of expertise. As educators, are we contributing to goal setting, implementation, and evaluation of nursing's contribution toward society's health? Are our educational programs consistent with these goals and will our graduates be prepared to practice accordingly?

The institutions or agencies to which we belong must also meet the test of accountability to their governing bodies and to society. What responsibilities do nurse teachers assume in participating in the formulation of philosophy and goals, in program planning and development, and in evaluating attainment of goals? To what extent are our own areas of control developed in concert with the goals of the institution?

The student, our direct consumer, is the pivotal person in our educational programs. Is the student getting the kind of program that is needed or is the program the one *we think* is needed or deserved? Are we asking the student to be an "abnormal eel" or a healthy vibrant learner? Where does the student fit into deliberations about program of studies? How well do we meet our contract with the learner?

Do our educational offerings stand the test of accountability? We as nurse teachers have been entrusted by society and by our profession with the responsibility to lead and to shape nursing. We are the gatekeepers of our profession, with the power to determine who enters the profession and to define the nature of nursing practice. How well are we using the power bestowed on us?

How well do we meet the test of accountability to ourselves? Are we authentic individuals? Have we formalized for ourselves values and beliefs that guide our actions? Are we true to those values, and are we real and genuine human beings?

The questions are raised here to remind nursing educators involved with the evaluation component of nursing programs that they must incorporate the concepts of relevance and responsibility for quality in any plan for accountability.

RELATIONSHIP OF BEHAVIORAL OBJECTIVES TO ACCOUNTABILITY

Throughout much of the history of education, educational objectives have been an integral part of program planning. For the most part, objectives have been generalized statements that did not lend themselves readily to operationalization in the curriculum nor to meaningful evaluation. Two movements have influenced educators to recognize the need for greater specificity and clarity in statements of objectives:

1. The development of programmed instruction.
2. Society's mandate for professional accountability.

The development of programmed instruction and instructional technology demonstrated the need for a more precise statement of objectives, so that the focal point of learning could be defined more sharply and the feedback evaluation made more specific.

Demand for accountability of educational endeavors now makes it necessary that student learning evaluation be related to instructional goals and efforts. This means that instructional accountability within our society has been shifted somewhat from the student to the instructor. This shift requires that clearly and precisely stated objectives must be used as a basis for determining accountability.

Behavioral objectives, unlike content objectives, are more amenable to evaluation. They are statements that describe the behavior the student is expected to exhibit as a result of one or more learning experiences. Emphasis on behavior means that evaluation is concerned with what the student does rather than on the "material covered," as is typical of content-oriented objectives.

The identification of behavior as the critical variable in the evaluation process arises from the concept of the learning process. Learning is described as a change in behavior as a result of "experiencing." Education is charged with expediting a student's learning by selecting experiences that foster the desired change in behavior. Therefore, selection of behaviors appropriate to a learning situation and their statement in measurable terms give direction to the learner's experiences and become the object of student evaluation.

INFLUENCE OF BEHAVIORAL OBJECTIVES ON THE TEACHING-LEARNING PROCESS

The teaching-learning process is a human transaction that has been taking place since the advent of man. Once limited to meeting survival needs within a sharply defined cultural group, it now relates not only to an individual's survival needs, but to the search for meaning in a complex pluralistic society. Pressures exerted on this transaction are constant, varied in intensity, and often dichotomous in nature. Each human being entering this transaction is surrounded by a particular life space or "bubble," which is unique to each and into which ideas, feelings, and values are selectively admitted.

The fragility of this transaction requires that educators provide the climate that assists participants toward mutual fulfillment. It is apparent in this complicated society that interactions among individuals depend on clear communication for effectiveness. This clarity of communication is most important when the teacher and learner meet, especially since a change in behavior is the expected outcome.

Behavioral objectives serve as a vital source of communication to all involved in this human transaction, without regard to whether concern is with a total nursing program or an individual learning experience. When the intent (expected behavior) is "on the table," there is little need for the learner to "psych out" the instructor. Since any given goal is clearly identified, all participants are able to channel their energies in the same direction. Not only does this result in maximal student learning efficiency, but it also promotes the climate of trust so essential to the teaching-learning process carried on as a shared enterprise.

Because our society is changing constantly, it is incumbent upon us, as educators, to assist the learner in accepting goal-directed learning as a life-long process. Since this implies accepting responsibility for one's own learning, our programs must provide sufficient learning experiences to internalize this value. Behavioral objectives offer students the opportunity to become self-directing. When the goals are clear, students can direct their own endeavors toward activities that will assist them in achieving these goals.

Behavioral objectives also discipline educators in their responsibilities as teachers. They force us to be clear and precise in communicating our intent. They make us select priorities in teaching and learning activities and help us to identify the trivia that may have been cluttering our educational endeavors. They require us to be well informed about *content* and *process*, as implied in the objectives. Most significantly, perhaps, they require us to meet our contract with the student. We state what is expected of the learner and are under contract to provide the kind of program that will facilitate the attainment of that behavior.

INFLUENCE OF BEHAVIORAL OBJECTIVES ON THE EVALUATION PROCESS

Evaluation has been a part of the teaching-learning process since humanity first became involved in it. At one time its focal point lay within a utilitarian framework; it answered the question: Is it useful? Today, there is not one focal point but many foci, as we deal with the complexity of an individual's response to the environment. Whereas historically educators made mental discipline the object of evaluation, today we are concerned with the learner as a whole being in an almost infinite variety of circumstances.

The evaluation process will be discussed further on in the book, but it is important to the discussion of objectives, at this point, to present one concept of evaluation. Nurse educators have asked repeatedly for a means for objective evaluation. The search has been pursued in many directions. (The impossible quest!) If one looks carefully at the word, one can see why objective evaluation is unattainable. The word e(valu)ation contains the word *value*, which connotes a personal choice.

Therefore anyone looking to behavioral objectives as a means of providing for *objective* evaluation will be disappointed. The very selection of the behaviors to be evaluated, whether selected by one person or many, is a personal choice.

Behavioral objectives, by their clarity, communicate the expected behavior signifying the learner's achievement. Thus the evaluator and the evaluatee know the behavior to be appraised. The element of the unexpected has been eliminated, and the learner does not need to direct energy toward trying to determine "what the test will be about." Although evaluation cannot be objective, it can be *fair*. Fairness in evaluation is a necessary prerequisite to a learning environment that fosters student growth.

Many nurse educators stress the need for nursing students to become self evaluating, as evaluation must be an on-going process throughout professional lifetimes. Because behavioral objectives are designed to foster measuring performance in terms of goals, the students possess a means for evaluating their own progress and organizing their efforts into relevant activities.

Behavioral objectives also discipline educators as to their evaluation responsibilities. They not only require us to state clearly what the student is to learn, but they also challenge us to evaluate that learning in appropriate ways. They also compel us to evaluate only what we have stated as our intent, thus precluding the inclusion of extraneous material. Of particular importance is adherence to evaluation of stated behavior. How often has a behavior been stated as *analyzing* a phenomenon, while the test question asks the student to *list* a certain number of characteristics of the phenomenon? Analyzing and listing are not the same intellectual behaviors.

ARGUMENTS AGAINST BEHAVIORAL OBJECTIVES

Behavioral objectives are not a panacea for all educational ills. Some educators do not even see them as significant to teaching and learning and regard their preparation as a pedagogic exercise. Most faculty have some objectives for their courses, but in many instances these objectives remain in the files, are available only on request, and have little relevancy to the actual learning situation.

Teachers of nursing have raised several arguments against behavioral objectives that are important for us to consider. There is no intent to deal with the issues in depth here, but perhaps this book will provide the rationale for further discussion. Three common arguments against behavioral objectives are:

1. They interfere with the freedom to learn and teach and thus stifle the creative process;

2. They require more time in development than is warranted by their effect in the program; and
3. Their preciseness is incompatible with a complex operation such as nursing.

The first argument is that behavioral objectives, by stating the anticipated result of the learning experience, restrict the freedom and creativity of the teacher and learner. This hypothesis arises, perhaps, from a misunderstanding of the use of objectives in a program of study. Behavioral objectives provide a framework from which a program, learning experience, or evaluation method can be developed. Structure, if relevant and flexible, does not stifle freedom but rather provides for it. One need only be a part of a blackout, such as New York experienced in 1965, to realize how necessary the structure of a network of traffic lights at street intersections is to the flow of traffic to a designated route or goal. Without the structure (lights), traffic halted at intersections until outside intervention became necessary. So, too, without the structure provided by behavioral objectives, learner and teacher may become immobilized at the intersection waiting for outside intervention. This delay may be costly in terms of time, and one cannot ignore the pressures of time on all individuals and the consequent responsibility of the educational endeavor to expedite the learning process.

Although the goal is defined, there is much opportunity for the teacher and learner to be creative in developing ways of meeting it. A stated goal does not mean that all learners and teachers must "march to the same drummer"; it does mean that once a goal has been established, participants are free to find their own drummers.

The second argument suggests that the development of behavioral objectives is a time-consuming process, the cost benefit of which does not justify the amount of time it requires. Perhaps one needs to consider the perspective one brings to the task of delineating objectives. Is it viewed as a mechanical task or is it a synthesizing process? Experience has indicated that as faculty members become involved in the process of developing behavioral objectives, they explore their own knowledge, values, and beliefs about the entire spectrum of teaching and learning; about nursing; about their society; and about themselves. Behavioral objectives really represent a synthesis of these explorations so that the follow-through of objectives into the program is expedited since much of the direction has already been charted.

In the third argument against the use of behavioral objectives, some faculty members suggest that the requirement for precision in behavioral objectives is inconsistent with the nature of nursing practice, which is a complex operation. The belief is that emphasis on particulars leads to compartmentalization of nursing practice; an unmanageable quantity of nursing behaviors; and emphasis on lower level behaviors. As one prepares behavioral objectives, it is important to realize that various developmental approaches are possible. Different forms need to be assessed for their appropriateness to a given situation. It may be that this concern of nurse-teachers has arisen because some think primarily of the form of behavioral objectives relevant to programmed instruction in which detail is essential. This matter will be dealt with in a later chapter, when the issue of generality and specificity in the preparation of behavioral objectives is explored. Behavioral objectives can be developed with respect for the multifaceted character of nursing practice, and when expressed within a taxonomy format, they challenge evaluation of the more complex levels of behavior.

OVERVIEW

This book supports the contention that carefully stated objectives are essential, providing direction for program planning and evaluation. It is not addressed to the total process of curriculum development and the many-faceted aspects of evaluation.

Goal-setting for any educational experience is as much a responsibility of the learner as of the teacher. Mutual respect for each other's objectives and a concerted effort to blend the two sets of objectives into a common set of goals provide for an educational experience that is both developmental and fulfilling.

In any program evaluation, accountability must be directed toward several components: the evaluation of student performance, the process used, and the rightness and completeness of goals. It must be recognized that some evaluation may not be directly related to a stated goal; that is, there may be goal-free evaluation as well as goal-directed evaluation.

The focus in this book, however, is between the behavioral objectives and evaluation. Its aim is to assist the nurse teacher in acquiring congruence between stated goals of instructional endeavor and the quality of strategies used to determine the degree to which the learner has attained the goals.

SUMMARY

Accountability for the quality of an educational endeavor has shifted from the learner to the teachers. In nursing, the teachers are accountable to the students, to society, to the institution providing the program, to the profession, and to themselves.

Behavioral objectives that identify the behavior the learner is expected to exhibit as a result of one or more learning experiences provide a basis for ascertaining accountability. These statements, in measurable terms, give direction to the learner's experiences and to the selection of strategies for determining learner attainment.

Behavioral objectives provide a means of communication among all involved in the learning experience, a focus for students' direction of their own learning, a discipline for educators in determining priorities, a contract between teacher and learner, and a means of fostering fairness in the evaluation process. Behavioral objectives are not a panacea for all educational ills. Some educators see them as interfering with the creative process and with the freedom to learn, consuming an unwarranted amount of time in their development, and incompatible with the complex process that is nursing.

RECOMMENDED READINGS

Chronister, J.L. Instructional Accountability in Higher Education. Educ. Rec. 51:171, Spring 1971.

Cohen, A.M. & Brawer, F. Measuring Faculty Performance. Washington, D.C.: American Association of Junior Colleges, 1969.

Eble, K.E. Professors as Teachers. San Francisco: Jossey-Bass, 1973.

Eble, K.E. Recognition and Evaluation of Teaching. Salt Lake City: Project to Improve College Teaching, 1970.

Gagne, R. Behavioral Objectives? Yes. Educ. Lead., 30:394, 1972.

Gerbner, G. Teacher Image and the Hidden Curriculum. Am. Schol., 42:66, Winter 1972-73.

Kibler, R., Barker L. & Miles, D. Behavioral Objectives and Instruction. Boston: Allyn and Bacon, 1970.

Kohnke, M.F. Do Nursing Educators Practice What Is Preached? Am. J. Nurs., 73:1571, 1973.

MacDonald J.B. & Wolfson, B.J. A Case Against Behavioral Objectives. Educ. Dig., 37:22, 1971.

Mager R.T. Preparing Educational Objectives. Palo Alto: Fearon, 1962.

Miller, W. Accountability Demands Involvement. Educ. Lead., 30:613, April 1972.

Morris, W.H. (ed). Effective College Teaching. Washington D.C.: American Council on Education, 1970.

Scriven, M. Pros and Cons About Goal-Free Evaluation. Evaluation Comment. J. Educ. Eval., 3:1, December 1972.

Tanner, D. Using Behavioral Objectives in the Classroom. New York: Macmillan, 1972.

Yager, S.J. Behavioral Objectives: Where and Where Not. Kappa Delta Pi Record 8:99, 1971.

2 Derivation of Behavioral Objectives

Two processes are involved in the development of behavioral objectives: one relates to their derivation and is addressed to the substance, the other relates to the writing and is addressed to the prescription for the technique. To insure significant input, participants in the development of these objectives should include representation from those directly involved with the program or learning experience, such as nurse-educators, consumers (nursing students, graduate nurses, patients, families, community groups), administrators, and experts in the subject matter.

The first process is a critical one in meeting the criteria of relevancy and responsibility for quality. Educational programs do not occur in a vacuum, but are always part of the teachers' and learners' total life experiences as well as those of the groups and society to which they belong. Failure to deal with this fact when developing behavioral objectives for a program leads to objectives limited in scope, inconsistent or unrealistic in behavioral expectations, and difficult if not impossible to evaluate. The derivation of substance then must include not only knowledge of subject matter of the discipline to be learned, but it must also include a knowledge of society and the profession as it relates to the program as well as the participants' values, attitudes, and beliefs about the nature of man, the learner, and the teaching-learning process in which all are involved.

Three steps are included in this derivation process. In the first step, participants explore their knowledges, values, beliefs, and attitudes relative to the seven areas depicted in Figure 2-1 (Source of Objectives Model):

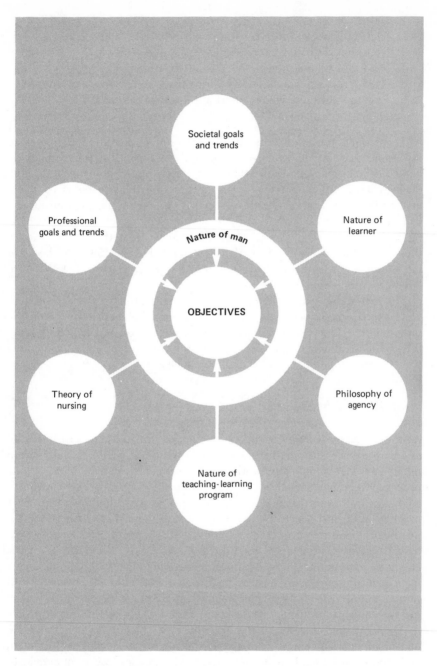

Figure 2-1. Source of Objectives Model.

1. Nature of man,
2. Societal goals and trends,
3. Professional goals and trends,
4. Nature of the learner,
5. Nature of the teaching-learning process,
6. Philosophy of the agency offering the programs, and
7. Theory of nursing.

There is no order of priority for these areas of investigation, thus they are represented as circular phenomena around the objective. Belief about the nature of man transcends all other areas, and thus is depicted as a circle through which all other areas transect. The questions to be asked in the exploration of these areas and the direction to be pursued in seeking answers will depend upon the nature of the program to be developed.

In the second step, the participants identify from their exploration of these areas the concepts, ideas, theories, and values pertinent to the learning situation. Synthesis is the last step of the process. Here the WHAT of behavioral objectives is clarified.

The rest of this chapter identifies some of the matters under each of these areas that have particular bearing on behavioral objectives for a nursing program. The identification is by no means extensive, but hopefully it will provide clues that will give direction to the thinking of groups concerned with the development of behavioral objectives.

NATURE OF MAN

An exposition of a group's concept of the nature of man is not only important as a basis for the teaching-learning interaction, but it is vital to the development of a conceptual framework for any program related to the helping process. Nursing (as well as medicine, ministry, social work, teaching) is among the groups identified as a helping profession; thus the nature of its practice is the service to human beings. Behaviors that characterize that practice depend on an individual's and group's concept of man.

Is man perceived within a dualistic framework, i.e., body and soul, mind and body, or is he perceived within the concept of unicity? Programs reflecting a dualistic concept are designed with an approach directed to each dualistic component, with some suggestion of synthesis, whereas programs reflecting the concept of unicity are designed with a single integrated approach.

Milhollan and Forisha (1972) identify two current diverse models of man—behavioristic and phenomenological—with which they feel individuals working with people need to be knowledgeable and aware of paradoxes.

The behavioristic orientation considers man to be a passive organism governed by stimuli supplied by the external environment. Man can be manipulated, that is, his behavior controlled through proper control of environmental stimuli.

The phenomenological orientation considers man to be the source of all acts. Man is essentially free to make choices in each solution. The focal point of his freedom is human consciousness. Behavior is thus only the observable expressions and consequences of an essentially private, internal world of being.[1]

The first model supports the concept of determinism and accepts the idea that man's behavior is predictable. Frankl (1963) denies the concept of pandeterminism and believes that the greatest force in man's life is the search for meaning as it relates to the self at any point in time. He states, ". . . Man is not fully conditioned and determined; he determines himself whether to give in to conditions or stand up to them. In other words, Man is self determining."[2] In reference to man's predictability, he states, " . . . every human being has the freedom to change at any instant. Therefore we can predict his future only within the large frame of a statistical survey referring to a whole group; the individual personality, however, remains essentially unpredictable."[3]

The two models certainly are not the only possible ones, but they are presented here to illustrate divergent concepts of the nature of man and his behavior; each would influence the type of behavioral outcome identified for a program of studies or a particular learning experience.

Exploration of the concept of man must include beliefs about man's response to stimuli in the internal and external environments. Stressors are inherent in all aspects of living, and questions need to be raised as to man's ability to adapt in the search for balance in life. Man's behavioral responses to stimuli represent a multiple, complex interaction in which harmony and accord are sought in terms of the values and needs at any time period in the individual's life. Individuals have resiliency and can adapt to disharmony. Beliefs about their potential for as well as their approaches to coping with or altering the environment influence behaviors deemed appropriate for a program in the helping professions.

SOCIETAL GOALS AND TRENDS

Man is a social creature constantly in interaction with the environment. He is both the initiator and the recipient of environmental forces that impinge on his daily life. He lives in an open system in which all parts are interrelated and in a constant state of flow.

Developers of behavioral objectives must come to terms with their ideas about the nature of society and the individual's relationship to that society, for society is the interface between the world and the individual. The objectives must reflect that society and their relationship to the goals, values, issues, and trends of that society.

The primary concern of nursing is with matters of health in a society. LeRiche and Milner (1971) define health as "the ability of an individual to function in a manner acceptable to himself and to the group of which he is a part."[4] This definition connotes a sociological emphasis rather than the usual pathological one of absence of disease. This concept then means that any aspect of society must be considered an influencing factor on an individual's health.

There are many issues in society about which developers of nursing programs need to be knowledgeable. Examples include questions relative to: Who receives medical care and how is it paid for? For whom is higher education available and how should it be supported? How is violence to be minimized in a highly industrialized society? How are the human rights of individuals to be guaranteed in a manner compatible with the Bill of Rights and the moral code? How is power to be used for the good of all? How are the resources of the world to be developed and used most effectively? How are the poor and disenfranchised to be accepted into the mainstream of society?

Trends, like issues, need to be scrutinized for their implications for the development of behavioral objectives. Current trends include: growing emphasis on nationalism; the internationalizing of currencies and industries; the greater mobility of individuals of varying cultures and nationalities; the rising middle class in many societies, especially in developing countries; the increasing equality for women in the labor force; the influence of third party payment in health care; the declaration of health as a human right; and the mobility of the population from the cities to the suburbs so that metropolises are being developed with no central governing force.

These are only a few of the issues and trends in the society of the 1980's, but their exploration and incorporation in objectives are essential to the relevancy of any nursing program. In a discussion group, a student stated that she perceived the nursing faculty's bedtime reading was nursing journals and textbooks. Seldom did class discussions relate to the outside world. Education carried on in such an insular manner contributes to a professional who is primarily technical rather than one who uses professional skills within the context of the needs of society in any particular period of time.

PROFESSIONAL GOALS AND TRENDS

One major criterion of a profession is that it be responsive to the needs of society. It must not only serve society, it must also provide leadership in implementing changes necessary for the health and welfare of that society. It both influences and is influenced by the goals, issues, and trends of the society. Although nursing is well identified by its service component, the report of the National Commission for the Study of Nursing and Nursing Education presents the view that nursing is "an occupation that fails in every characteristic to achieve the status of a full profession, despite the fact that its best practitioners are professional in every sense of the word. It is an occupation that has never controlled its own destiny, but has suffered severe consequences when it has failed to meet the demands imposed by society."[5]

Nursing represents the largest group within the health care system and has the potential for markedly influencing the quality of health care given in this society. Its goals must be clearly defined and a course of action zealously pursued, if it is to be identified as a viable and essential profession within the health care system.

Any nursing program, whether for the practitioner or the prospective practitioner, must be designed to be consistent with these goals and courses of action, and must address itself to issues and trends affecting the profession in pursuit of its goals.

In the 1980's the nature of nursing practice and role relationship with other health professions will continue to be critical issues. Nursing practice is increasingly shifting its focus from disease to health. This shift is evidenced by the emphasis on primary care function relating to health screening, continuity of care, and health education. As medical technology and automation continue to make inroads in the therapeutic and diagnostic aspects of care, nursing is called upon to assume greater responsibility for humanizing care and must be prepared to make value judgments on ethical and moral issues inherent in modern-day practice. Not only must nursing evolve its practice according to changing societal needs, it must also develop and utilize systematic approaches to quality control to assure that its practice meets prescribed standards.

Much is said about the need for interdisciplinary collaboration to insure best use of health resources, but true collaboration, which is a shared process of decision-making, is still relatively rare. As demands for health care increase, health team members will need to be less role conscious (a territorial connotation), and more problem oriented, that is, the person who is ultimately responsible for meeting the health need at any moment is the one designated by preparation and competency rather than by role definition or position on the team.

The changing nature of practice must evolve from the findings of research and must be developed in educational programs, using a nursing rather than a medical model. Objectives must be expressed in behavioral terms compatible with this evolving process and representative of the varied nursing competencies essential for its implementation.

Nursing must also address itself to identifying the types of practitioners needed to meet this developing practice, and to identifying the types of educational programs indicated. The educational program is the gatekeeper of the profession, as such it has the responsibility to determine WHO will enter as well as the WHAT and HOW dimensions of the preparation of future practitioners.

As objectives are developed for these programs, participants must be knowledgeable about other movements that affect nursing, such as: requirements for entry into professional nursing practice; changing patterns of state licensure for practice; identification of newer meanings in the concept of accreditation; approaches to all aspects of credentialing; a shift in governmental participation away from health care so that support for educational programs has been reduced; emphasis on continuing education as a criterion for licensure; extension of nursing's resources and facilities to members of minority groups; and the use of the profession's leadership within the power structure at all levels of government. Nursing's response to these movements and its willingness to be held accountable for its actions will determine its future within the society. Program developers must prepare practitioners who exhibit behaviors indicative of wisdom in decision-making, problem-solving in health matters, and responsibility for accountability to self, clients, and society.

NATURE OF THE LEARNER

Regardless of the educational endeavor, the learner is the focal point, for it is the learner's behavior that is to be developed according to stated goals. Since the program is designed for the student, participants in program development must be knowledgeable about the goals, values, interests, and learning style of the learner, in addition to the usual demographic data about the social, cultural, and academic background.

The kinds of data one seeks about the learner originate from basic beliefs about the learner and reflect beliefs about the nature of man. Is the learner to be controlled or is the learner to become a self controlling individual with impulses and desires ordered by intelligence? Is the learner someone to whom things are done or someone who does things?

If educational programs are viewed within a developmental context, they start where the students are and lead them toward greater use of their potential. Therefore knowledge of students at the point of entry into an educational experience is essential if behavioral objectives are to be realistic. It is important that faculty guard against projecting their own prejudicial or value connotations when interpreting these data. The homogeneity of nursing students in terms of life style, social and economic background, educational experience, values, and residence orientation has given way to diversity as various ethnic and socioeconomic groups become involved.

As nursing educational opportunities are made available to groups in our society that were previously disenfranchised from higher education, nursing has become an avenue of upward mobility for many individuals. For some, nursing provides the opportunity for career employment, as the changing socioeconomic scene places limitations on employment possibilities in some career fields. Motivations for entering nursing and for participating in programs of study beyond the basic preparation are varied and complex. The diversity of motivating forces in any group of nursing learners must be recognized by program planners.

Age is certainly a critical variable today as the adult learner appears on the nursing scene in more frequent numbers in schools of nursing, in continuing education programs, and in community groups with which nurses are engaged in a teaching-learning situation. Diverse motivations are present in this group. For some the opportunity of a career choice can be realized and entry into the mainstream of American society is possible. For others a change in career becomes an option for synthesizing a life style with values and desires for service to man and his society. All nursing programs feel the impact of these adult learners as the concept of life-long learning becomes accepted in practice.

Nursing has not yet significantly increased the number of males among its practitioners but these numbers also are changing. Men with experience in the medical corps are seeking opportunities to relate the practice skills they learned to a health career, such as nursing. The expanding role of nursing, the variety of opportunities for practice, and the acceptance of men in our society in the nurturance role should increase male participation in the profession.

We also see heterogeneity in the educational experience represented by students with limited educational preparation and students with all degrees of experience up to and including graduation from college. We further note the demise or lessening of the importance of nurses' residence as more students become commuters who may be working part-time or have family responsibilities.

Many of these characteristics are found in staff education programs, particularly as various types of practitioners engage in meeting the nursing needs of individuals.

In any event more attention needs to be paid to the values, interests, attitudes, and aspirations of the learners in every program. Chickering (1969) reminds us that ". . . colleges and universities will be educationally effective only if they reach the students 'where they live,' only if they connect significantly with those concerns of central importance to their students."[6] This comment is relevant to any program of studies and challenges the developers of behavioral objectives to really *know* their students.

NATURE OF THE TEACHING-LEARNING PROCESS

The teaching-learning process is the mode through which behavioral objectives are reached, and thus one's perspective of this process greatly influences the substance of the objectives. Since this process is viewed as a human transaction, one's concept obviously becomes dependent on one's belief of the nature of man.

There are numerous theories of learning based on various assumptions about man, the nature of knowledge, and the process by which one learns. A theory of instruction that is predictive and normative has yet to be developed and Brunner (1968) notes that there is no theory of instruction that can serve as a guide to pedagogy; in its place is primarily a body of maxims.[7]

A teacher operates within the framework of a theory of learning, whether or not it can be verbalized, because the teaching activity would otherwise be purposeless and obscure. The approaches to teaching and the expectations of a learner and teacher reflect this theory. If the objectives are to be substantive, however, teachers must conceptualize the teaching-learning process in terms meaningful to themselves so that they have a framework for determining actions and evaluating results.

Various classifications of learning theorists exist, but in general they may be identified as associationists, conditionists, behaviorists, cognitive field theorists, and phenomenological theorists (often called Third Force). Explorations of the learning process through the biophysical mechanisms are now underway. All theorists basically accept a concept of learning as a change in behavior through experience. The dimension of experience is critical in differentiating the behavioral change due to learning from that due to maturation.

The two most widely diverse concepts of man—behavioristic and phenomenological—form a basis for the two prominent theories in educational practices in current favor. In the behavioristic model, one accepts the teaching process as a controlling one in which techniques are designed so that reinforcement contingencies, the relationships between behavior and the consequences of that behavior, are arranged. The reinforcement is positive and avoids any semblance of aversion control. B. F. Skinner (1972), one of the most noted members of the behavioristic school of thought, believes that "man's struggle for freedom is not due to a will to be free, but to certain behavioral processes characteristic of the human organism, the chief effect of which is the avoidance of or an escape from so-called 'aversion features of the environment.' "[8]

The phenomenological school of thought sees man as basically good, with much potential to be better. The teaching process with this perspective is a facilitating one in which the individual develops an identity and those inner forces that bring about a response. It recognizes needs as energizing forces in learning and calls for significant meaningful experiential learning. Rogers[9] (1969) identifies five characteristics of this type of learning:

1. Personal involvement,
2. Self initiated,
3. Pervasive,
4. Evaluated by the learner,
5. Its essence is meaning.

Dewey (1963) sees experimental learning as being in harmony with growth.[10]

Reinforcement is intrinsic and freedom to learn is equated with a climate of trust, authenticity, and intelligent risk taking. Dewey recognizes aversive controls as impediments to freedom, but he states that "the only freedom that is of enduring importance is freedom of intelligence, that is to say, freedom of observation and judgment exercised in behalf of purposes that are intrinsically worthwhile."[11] It is the business of teaching to facilitate that freedom of intelligence, and this must be accomplished through experience in choosing between alternatives and learning to learn in preparation for making choices in a world of ambiguities and rapid change.

The cognitive field theory of learning is also relevant to nursing practice, for it concerns an individual's knowledge of self and the surrounding environment. It identifies learning as the process by which one gains new insights, by which one changes perceptions. Milhollan and Forisha see congruence between Lewin's field theory and Rogers' phenomenological theory in terms of their identification as a human science. Three characteristics of Lewin's field theory,[12] which support this psychology of human science, are:

1. A field is considered to be the totality of coexisting facts—external and internal—which are conceived as mutually interdependent;
2. Behavior is a function of this field or life space which exists at the moment behavior occurs; and
3. Analysis begins with the situation as a whole (experience as it is given).

Teaching then is holistic rather than additive; learning takes place through problem-solving as new perceptions are gained; reinforcement is through inner experience of the organism as it gives meaning to the environment.

As indicated in this discussion, the teaching process is very much related to the theoretical framework of learning, which people evolve for themselves. Teaching, however, is a process in its own right and has its own qualities. Gibran[13] (1968) conceptualizes teaching as follows:

Then said a teacher, Speak to us of teaching: And he said: No man can reveal to you aught, but that which already lies half asleep in the dawning of your knowledge.

The teacher who walks in the shadow of the temple, among his followers, gives not of his wisdom but rather of his faith and his lovingness.

If he is indeed wise he does not bid you enter the house of his wisdom, but rather leads you to the threshold of your own mind.

In this concept, teaching is viewed as a guiding of the learning experiences of students so that they become involved in their own learning.

Nouwen[14] (1971) identifies two types of teaching, violent and redemptive. Violent teaching is seen as:

1. Competitive, with fear the dominant feeling tone;
2. Unilateral, in which the teacher is all knowing and strong while the student is ignorant and weak; and
3. Alienating, in which the student is directed outward away from the self and a direct relationship to the future.

In contrast, redemptive teaching is viewed as:

1. Evocative, where student and teacher evoke each other's potentials;
2. Bilateral, where student and teacher are both teachers and learners in an open environment; and
3. Actualizing, by which the student's future becomes present in the learning situation, and the classroom becomes the setting for creative interchange and experience in identifying models for life styles in the modern world.

This presentation of the teaching-learning process is obviously a limited one for such a complex process, but hopefully it will help nurse teachers to conceptualize the process for themselves so that they will have a basis for determining the types of behavioral outcomes expected of the learner.

PHILOSOPHY AND PURPOSE OF AGENCY OFFERING THE PROGRAM

A program of studies operates within the framework of a specific agency which has its own social and educational philosophy. As part of that agency's system, the educational program must have objectives which are consistent with the expressed philosophy and purpose of that agency. Tyler (1950) perceives the educational and social philosophy of a school as a screen for selecting objectives most salient to the institution's beliefs and values. Behaviors inconsistent with the philosophy are discarded.[15]

The same concept applies to staff development programs in health agencies. The agency's philosophy of nursing practice and its expressed commitment to staff development for its practitioners serve as a guide for formulating objectives for that program.

When a conflict occurs between the desire for a particular behavioral objective and the need to implement a philosophy not supportive of this behavior, the solution must be found in either changing the philosophy or discarding the objective. Faculty may want to express behavioral objectives in the higher cognitive skills, but if the philosophy of the school supports open admission, levels of behaviors must be geared to the highest level most students can achieve.

Thus, in the process of developing objectives, one must identify behaviors suggested by the philosophy of the agency and aim toward developing them in the program.

THEORY OF NURSING

Program developers in a profession refer to their theory of practice to aid them in identifying appropriate behaviors. This theory serves to focus the goals of the practice, to define its boundaries or parameters, and to describe its nature in relation to the clients served, the types of problems with which it is concerned, its methodology, and the value base upon which it rests.

Nursing, a theoretically based practice discipline, requires a theory of nursing practice. Argyris and Schön (1974) define a theory of practice: "A theory of practice consists of a set of interrelated theories of action that specify for the situations of the practice, the actions that will, under relevant assumptions, yield intended consequences. Theories of practice usually contain theories of intervention, that is, theories of action aimed at enhancing effectiveness; these may be differentiated according to roles in which intervention is attempted—for example, counseling and teaching."[16] A theory of practice is essential for directing the endeavors of a profession. Without a theory base, a practice is subject to inconsistency, irrationality, and unpredictability as it becomes self-serving. These characteristics result primarily because its derivation is from intuition, imitation or a professional mystique that surrounds some of its "successful" members rather than from a theoretical basis.

The practice theory then becomes the root of the profession which serves its practitioners, its educators, and its researchers. It is the WHAT.

It is generally accepted that nursing theory is evolving as research in nursing practice generates the new knowledge upon which the practice is based. Research establishing the congruency of theories and concepts from related disciplines in the sciences and humanities to the practice of nursing is underway and suggests that a nursing practice theory will indeed be a synthesis of relevant theories and concepts from these disciplines.

During the past decade, nursing educators, researchers, and practitioners have been involved in the development of conceptual models of nursing practice which seeks to provide the framework served by a theory, namely: focusing the goals of practice; defining its boundaries; and describing its nature in relation to clients served, the types of problems with which it is concerned, its methodology, and the value base on which it rests. This pattern or model, however, differs from a theoretical one in that it is a description of the practice since many of its components are derived from experience, intuition, and empirical data rather than from data supplied by research.

This model (Reilly, 1975) says what appears to be; it does not say what is, which a theoretical model would do. Since it is a conceptual representation of reality, it is not reality. A theoretical model does constitute reality since it has a scientifically supported base.[17] Although the conceptual model is not reality, it must be congruent with accepted practice as defined by the profession at a particular point in its development. A conceptual model then is descriptive rather than predictive.

Rogers (1970) sees the nursing conceptual system as a new emergent: "The unifying principle and hypothetical generalizations basic to nursing seek to describe, explain, and predict about the phenomena central to nursing's purpose—MAN."[18]

Nursing, in its development toward identifying its own practice as distinct unto itself and different from that of other health disciplines, is seeking its own nursing model. This developmental process which identifies nursing practice within a holistic view of man demands a model which is more encompassing than the medical model, which has been used by nurses since the evolution of scientific knowledge and technology brought disease control and intervention within the medical domain.

Several components of a nursing theory have already been identified through practice which can be incorporated into a conceptual framework:

1. Nature of man and his total being (internal and external environment) through the entire life span.
2. Society, its systems, values, and norms as man interfaces with it.
3. The dynamics of the process by which an individual maintains integrity and wholeness during the continuous interaction and sharing of energy and matter with the external environment.
4. Health definitions in terms of meaning to an individual, group, or society.
5. Health care delivery system as it relates to both individuals and the greater society.

6. Morals and ethics inherent in human interactions.

The question before nursing is how are these components related? What matrix can be woven from these components and their interaction with nursing so that a framework exists that is nursing practice?

A conceptual model of nursing practice must have a unifying concept to which all components are related. There are several classifications of nursing practice models, each determined by the nature of the unifying component.

1. Systems model
    Stress adaptation
    Behavioral system
    Social system
    Community health (health care system)
    Kinship
    Self care
2. Developmental model (longitudinal)
    Erikson's stages of man
    Sullivan's interpersonal theory.
    Interpersonal relationship
    Sociocultural–socialization
    Role theory
    Health-illness continuum
3. Life processes (energy producing)

Currently there is no conceptual model accepted by nursing. Nursing theorists are presently engaged in theory building as research seeks more definitive data relative to the substance of the practice of nursing. The behavioral objectives of any program must reflect the conceptual framework accepted by the faculty responsible for the program.

SUMMARY

Derivation of the substance of objectives involves carefully exploring at least seven areas: the nature of man; societal goals and trends; professional goals and trends; the nature of the learner; the nature of the teaching-learning process; philosophy and goals of the agency; and theories of nursing. All are interrelated, yet each has its own function, independent of the total, and has special tasks to perform. The challenge to the developers of behavioral objectives is to identify relevant concepts of each area and then synthesize these into a unifying substance, suggesting the behaviors indicated. All areas must be explored if objectives are to meet the criteria of relevancy and accountability.

REFERENCES

1. Milhollan, F. & Forisha, B. From Skinner to Rogers. Lincoln, Nebraska: Professional Educators Publication, 1972.
2. Frankl, V. Man's Search for Meaning. New York: Washington Square Press, 1963, p. 206.
3. *Idem.* p. 20.
4. LeRiche, W.H. & Milner, J. Epidemiology as Medical Ecology. Edinburgh, London: Churchill Livingstone, 1971, p. 82.
5. Lysaught, J.P. (ed). An Abstract for Action. New York: McGraw-Hill, 1970 (Blakiston), p. 163.
6. Chickering, A.W. Education and Identity. San Francisco: Jossey-Bass, 1969, p. 3.
7. Brunner, J.S. Toward a Theory of Instruction. Cambridge, Mass.: Belknap Press of Harvard University Press, 1968, p. 31.
8. Skinner, B.F. Beyond Freedom and Dignity. New York: Random House, 1972, p. 39.
9. Rogers, C. Freedom to Learn. Columbus, Ohio: Charles E. Merrill, 1969, p. 5.
10. Dewey, J. Experience and Education. New York: Macmillan, 1963, p. 27.
11. *Idem.* p. 61.
12. Milhollan, F. & Forisha, B. *op cit.* p. 93.
13. Gibran, K. The Prophet (2nd ed.). New York: Alfred A. Knopf, 1968, p. 56.
14. Nouwen, H.J.M. Creative Ministry. Garden City, New York: Doubleday, 1971, pp. 4-14.
15. Tyler, R.W. Basic Principles of Curriculum and Instruction. Chicago: University of Chicago, 1950, p. 22.
16. Argyris, C. & Schön, D. Theory in Practice: Increasing Professional Effectiveness. San Francisco: Jossey-Bass, 1974, p. 6.
17. Reilly, D. Why a Conceptual Framework? Nurs. Outl., 23:566, September 1975.
18. Rogers, M. An Introduction to the Theoretical Basis of Nursing. Philadelphia: F.A. Davis, 1970, p. 111.

RECOMMENDED READINGS

American Academy of Nursing: Models for Health Care Delivery: Now and For the Future, Kansas City, Mo.: American Academy of Nursing, 1975.
Auger, J.R. Behavioral Systems and Nursing, Englewood Cliffs, N.J.: Prentice-Hall Inc., 1976.
Ausbel, D. Historical Overview of Theoretical Trends. In Eliot, J. (ed): Human Development and Cognitive Processes. New York: Holt, Rinehart and Winston Inc., 1971.
Bevis, E.O. Curriculum Building in Nursing: A Process. (2nd ed). St. Louis: Mosby, 1978.
Bigge, M. Learning Theories for Teachers, New York: Harper and Row, 1964.
Brown, E.L. Nursing Reconsidered: A Study of Change (Part I). Philadelphia: Lippincott, 1970.
Brunner, J.S. Toward a Theory of Instruction. Cambridge, Mass.: Belknap Press of Harvard University Press, 1968.
Byrne, M.L. & Thompson, L.F. Key Concepts for the Study and Practice of Nursing. St. Louis: Mosby, 1972.
Clayton, T.E. Teaching and Learning. Englewood Cliffs, N.J.: Prentice-Hall, 1965.
Dacey, J. New Ways to Learn: The Psychology of Education. Stamford, Conn.: Greylock Pub., 1976.

DeMott, B., McDermott, J.J., & Mann, R.: Teaching, the Uncertain Profession. Change, 1972, 4:48.

deTornyay, R. Strategies for Teaching Nursing. New York: Wiley, 1971.

Downs, F.S. & Fleming, J.W. Issues in Nursing Research. New York: Appleton-Century-Crofts, 1979.

Dunn, H.L. High Level Wellness. Arlington, Va.: Beatty, 1973.

Eble, K. Professors as Teachers. San Francisco: Jossey-Bass, 1973.

Eble, K. The Craft of Teaching. San Francisco: Jossey-Bass, 1976.

————Entry Into Nursing Practice: Proceedings of the National Conference. Kansas City, Mo.: American Nurses Association, 1978.

Erikson, E.H. Identity Youth and Crisis. New York: W.W. Norton, 1968.

Frank, E. Teaching Without Learning. Nurs. For., 1970, 9:131.

Frankena, W.K. Philosophy of Education. New York: Macmillan, 1965.

Goble, F. The Third Force. New York: Pocketbooks, 1971.

Henderson, A.D. The Innovative Spirit. San Francisco: Jossey-Bass, 1970.

Hill, W.F. Learning. A Survey of Psychological Interpretation. Scranton: Chandler, 1971.

Hodgman, E.C. A Conceptual Framework to Guide Nursing Curriculum. Nurs. For., 1973, 12:111.

Jourard, S. The Transparent Self. New York: Van Nostrand-Reinhold, 1971.

King, I.M. Toward a Theory for Nursing. New York: Wiley, 1971.

Maccoby, M. A Psychoanalytic View of Learning. Change, 1971, 3:32.

May, R.L. Man's Search for Himself. New York: W.W. Norton, 1953.

McAttee, P. The Human Side of Curriculum Development. Nurs. For., 1969, 8:144.

Murphy, J. Theoretical Issues in Professional Nursing. New York: Appleton-Century-Crofts, 1971.

Nursing Development Conference Group. Concept Formalization in Nursing. Process and Product. Boston: Little, Brown, 1973.

Reynolds, P.D. Primer in Theory Construction, Indianapolis: Bobbs-Merrill Educational Publ., 1977.

Riehl, J.R. & Roy, Sr. C. Conceptual Models for Nursing Practice (2nd ed.). New York: Appleton-Century-Crofts, 1980.

Rogers, M. An Introduction to the Theoretical Basis of Nursing. Philadelphia: F.A. Davis, 1970.

Roy, Sr. C. Introduction to Nursing: An Adaptation Model. Englewood Cliffs, N.J.: Prentice-Hall, Inc., 1976.

Sanford, N. (ed). The American College. New York: Wiley, 1962.

Schein, E.N. Professional Education: Some New Directions. New York: McGraw-Hill Books Co., 1972.

Shields, M. A Model For a Curriculum Goal. Nurs. Outl., 1972, 20:782.

Shostrom, E. Man, The Manipulator. New York: Bantam, 1968.

Silva, M.C. The Educational Process in Perspective. Nurs. For., 1972, 2:47.

Sutterly, D.C. & Donnelly, G.F. Perspectives in Human Development. Philadelphia:Lippincott, 1973.

Vaillot, Sr. M.C. Nursing Theory, Levels of Nursing and Curriculum Development. Nurs. For., 1970, 9:234.

Williamson, J.A. (ed). Current Perspectives in Nursing Education: The Changing Scene. St. Louis, Mo.: Mosby, 1976.

3 Development of Behavioral Objectives

After the substance of the objectives has been identified by exploring the seven areas discussed in the previous chapter and after synthesis of their common elements, program developers must write behavioral objectives that truly communicate the intent of the planners. Objectives are tools that guide all activities of the program designers and participants in the educational endeavor. Formulation of these objectives represents the conscious choice of the planners and must be expressed in terms that are clear to all who are involved in implementing them.

As planners develop behavioral objectives, they must recognize that behaviors are expressed in relation to students, not teachers. The educational endeavor is geared toward change in the learner's behavior and it is this change that is to be evaluated. The real purpose is not to assay what the teacher does. That is not to say that the teacher's behavior is not also subject to change during this academic endeavor and indeed, if a redemptive interaction is occurring, the teacher also will be a learner. The teacher might set up behavioral objectives for him- or herself as a tool for self-evaluation. However, program developers devise behavioral objectives addressed to those changes indicated for the learner.

There are two dimensions to the preparation of behavioral objectives. One relates to the technique of writing objectives and will be discussed in this chapter. The second is concerned with ordering behaviors according to the complexity of each. This latter will be developed in subsequent chapters dealing with the concept of taxonomy.

COMPONENTS OF A BEHAVIORAL OBJECTIVE

The development of behavioral objectives represents a very inexact field of endeavor and, indeed, the literature on this subject reflects various points of view. It is important to recognize that there are several formulas for writing objectives, and that the use intended for behavioral objectives determines the choice of an appropriate formula. Review of the literature suggests two major classifications for behavioral objectives—specific and general. The prescription for each of these types will be presented and their meaning and use discussed.

Specific Behavioral Objectives

The prescription for this type of objective was proposed by behaviorists and other educationists, particularly in response to the necessity for behavioral objective specificity in program planning.

In general there are four elements in the objective:

1. Description of the learner.
2. Description of the behavior the learner will exhibit to demonstrate that competence has been attained.
3. Description of conditions under which the learner will demonstrate competence. The description notes specific restrictions imposed.
4. Statement of standard of performance expected to indicate excellence.

EXAMPLE: Given a slide tape in which a man and a woman read Rod McKuen's poem, "Knowing When to Leave," the nursing student will identify, in writing, the difference in communication between men and women in terms of pitch, voice, enunciation, and facial expressions.

ANALYSIS OF THE BEHAVIORAL OBJECTIVE

1. Description of the learner	Nursing student
2. Description of the behavior	Identify in writing communication differences between men and women.
3. Description of conditions	Given a slide tape of a woman and man reading the Rod McKuen poem, "Knowing When to Leave."
4. Statement of standard	Four differences must be discussed: pitch, voice, enunciation, facial expression.

General Behavioral Objectives

The prescription was suggested by Tyler (1950) and others. Kibler, Barker, and Miles (1970) call this type of objective informational.[1] Basically there are three elements in this type of behavioral objective.

1. Description of the learner.
2. Statement of the kind of behavior the learner will exhibit to demonstrate competence has been attained.
3. Statement of the kind of content to which behavior relates. (Kibler et al. combine 2 and 3.)

EXAMPLE: The nursing student distinguishes differences between male and female patterns of communication.

ANALYSIS OF THE BEHAVIORAL OBJECTIVE

1. Description of the learner   Nursing student

2. Description of the behavior   Distinguish differences

3. Statement of content   Male and female patterns of communication

GENERALITY VS. SPECIFICITY

The two approaches to writing behavioral objectives have similarities and differences. In essence, they are similar in two fundamental aspects: They agree that the nature of the learner must be specified, and they agree that the objective must be expressed in terms of behavior. The difference occurs in the desirability of including specific information about conditions of learning and criteria for performance acceptance. As one analyzes dissimilarities between these two approaches, it is important that judgments not be made as to which is the better. Rather, each type should be considered in terms of the situations in which it could be used most effectively.

Tanner (1972) sees the present emphasis on the specificity of behavioral objectives as being derived from the operant conditioning concept of the Behavioristic School, represented by Skinner and his followers.[2] As discussed previously in this book, teaching, as perceived by the Behavioristic School, is based on the theory that contingencies of reinforcement need to be arranged and that learning is an additive process. Skinner (1968) expresses this view when he says, "The whole process of becoming competent in any field must be divided into a very large number of very small steps, and reinforcement must be contingent upon an accomplishment of each step."[3]

Tanner also sees specificity as limited to the lower cognitive process development of the learner, and states, "Because behavioral objectives are so explicitly defined they tend to be limited to the lower cognitive process of recalling specifics and knowing the ways and means of dealing with specifics."[4]

Exploration of the nature of knowledge from an epistemologic perspective is not in order in this book, but there are some considerations that have a direct bearing on writing behavioral objectives. Some educators refer to the process of recalling *information,* while others may refer to the process of recalling *knowledge.* Discrimination between these two terms may connote a very different meaning to the intent of the objective. Information may be perceived as facts, laws, theories, and specifics known to the population in general or within specific groups. Knowledge, however, is personal to the learner and is obtained only after learning has occured. In this context, information becomes one of the tools by which the learner gains knowledge.

Dewey and Whitehead add another critical dimension to the concept of knowledge—that is, utilization. Dewey (1961) defines knowledge as "perception of the connections of an object which determine its applicability in a given situation," and describes an ideally perfect knowledge as "such a network of interconnections that any past experience would offer a point of advantage from which to get at the problem presented in a new experience."[5]

Whitehead (1958) states, "Education with inert ideas is not only useless; it is above all things harmful."[6] He further describes what he means by utilizing ideas. "I mean relating it to that stream, compounded of sense, perceptions, feelings, hopes, desires, and mental activities adjusting thought to thought, which forms our life."[7]

Boulding (1961), as he differentiates between the image and the message, postulates that a highly learned process of interpretation and acceptance influences the way a message is received. He states, ". . . what this means is that for any individual or group or organization, there are no such things as 'facts.' There are only messages filtered through a changeable value system."[8] Boulding's organic theory of knowledge is based on the following two propositions:

1. Knowledge is that which somebody or something knows; and that without a knower, knowledge is an absurdity.
2. Growth of knowledge is the growth of an organic structure, meaning it follows principles of growth and development similar to those with which we are familiar in complex organization.[9]

These concepts of knowledge connote a dynamic quality greatly influenced by the learner's perceptions, which represent integrated experiences and are available for meeting the exigencies of life. It is not information, but rather the personalization of information that is useful. If there is growth in knowledge, then its direction is developmental, not accumulative.

Emphasis on specificity contrasts with the view of generality. Tyler supports the concept of generality when he states, "I tend to view objectives as general modes of reaction to be developed, rather than specific habits to be acquired."[10] He further states, "So far as behavioral aspect of objectives is concerned, the problem of generality and specificity is one of obtaining the level of generality desired and what is in harmony with what we know about the psychology of learning."[11]

Bloom et al. (1965) believe that specifics are best learned in relation to general abstractions. They state, "When learning takes place in this way, it is possible for an individual who remembers the generalization to proceed relatively easily to some specifics subsumed under generalization. On the other hand, generalization or abstraction are relatively difficult to learn unless they are related to appropriate concrete phenomenon."[12]

The question program developers must deal with is the desirability of stressing generalities or specifics in any particular learning situation.

Several other concerns are relevant to the issue of specificity and generality. One relates to implications for the teaching-learning process. The specificity concepts imply a model of man as mechanistic and automatic, whereas the generality implies a model of man as an open system. The specific behavioral objective provides all the "givens" and controls the activities of learner and teacher. All must reach the goal through the same route, and all must be evaluated by the same method and according to the same criteria.

A general behavioral objective, on the other hand, clarifies expected outcome, but leaves students and faculty free to determine the path to the objective and the approach to evaluation. This enables the teaching-learning process to become personal, human, and facilitating, since the learner's needs, interests, and capabilities can be considered in reaching the expressed outcome. Since all the "givens" are not provided, the creative potentials of the teacher and learner are aroused and have the opportunity for development. Furthermore, since the focus of participants is not limited, all are able to identify and capitalize on collateral learnings that often occur because one's total being is involved in any human interaction.

Many criteria for performance, as stated in specific behavioral objectives, include a time or other quantifiable factor, such as "two out of three times." Unless time is a critical variable in a skill, to include it ignores the fact that among as well as within individuals a wide range of time is needed to master a task. Quantifying the outcome, except for specific learning tasks, is less desirable than qualifying the outcome.

One realistic and practical concern, however, has particular relevancy if specific behavioral objectives are to be used widely in nursing. This concern relates to the tremendous numbers of specific behavioral objectives necessary for the complex operation of nursing. Tanner is concerned with this problem when he states, "The ultraspecificity of such behaviors would require each teacher and student to work with hundreds of thousands of explicit objectives."[13]

USE OF SPECIFIC AND GENERAL BEHAVIORAL OBJECTIVES

From previous discussions, it is apparent that a different premise underlies each type of behavioral objective, both specific and general, and that uses for each type vary.

In nursing programs, specific behavioral objectives would seem to be most applicable to learning experiences incorporated in programmed instruction. They would also be most helpful in designating outcomes of individual learning experiences in the practice setting or classroom.

General behavioral objectives would be used most frequently to communicate the intent of programs to others interested in them. As stated earlier, Kibler et al. refer to these as informational objectives and suggest their use for a curriculum, a course, a weekly unit, or a daily lesson plan.[14] This form of behavioral objective would find widespread use in nursing instruction for communicating expected outcomes of programs. Students would be informed as to expected behaviors and thus direct their energies toward expectations; teachers would be able to relate their own teaching to past and future learning of students; and administrators would have a clear perspective of the intent of the program so that they could facilitate the environment and resources necessary for attainment of objectives.

POINTS IN WRITING BEHAVIORAL OBJECTIVES

Many books and articles have been written about the technique for writing behavioral objectives. References included at the end of this chapter contain suggestions for sources this writer found helpful. A few major points about technique are, however, germane. In principle, objectives should be written clearly, concisely, and in the vernacular of the learner.

Behavioral Terms

The critical aspect of any behavioral objective is the word selected to indicate expected behavior from an educational experience. A behavioral term is one that is considered by some to be observable and measurable. Behavior generally is construed to be any action of an individual that can be seen, felt, or heard by another person. A concept of action implies psychomotor involvement. Kibler et al. warn us about overemphasizing the action component of objectives when they state, "Cognitive and affective objectives are concerned with characteristics of thinking and feeling which are themselves not directly observable. States of affection and acts of cognition are *inferred* from psychomotor acts." As an illustration, they add: "We do not see a person analyze a poem; we see or hear a report of his analysis."[15] Thus the significant characteristic of the behavioral term is its measurability.

Some words commonly found in objectives, however, imply no action. The terms *understanding, knowledge,* and *appreciation* are nonactive and provide no direction for program development or qualitative assessment. Indeed, the term *understanding* can represent any of a wide range of cognitive processes, from simple to complex. Since the major function of behavioral objectives is communication, the terms used must be defined by the individuals concerned so that all interpret the words similarly and use them consistently with the same intent. Chapter 4, page 64 provides a list of suggested action verbs appropriate for each level of the taxonomy for the three domains of learning.

One Behavior Per Objective

A behavioral objective expresses the intended outcome, not outcomes, of a learning experience and must be amenable to credentialing. One pattern of writing behavioral objectives frequently encountered shows that two or more behaviors have been included in one objective. This practice makes it difficult to evaluate the outcome, for the learner may attain one behavior but not the others. For example, the following behavioral objective includes two cognitive behaviors:

> *The nursing student identifies and analyzes phenomena in the patient's environment that influence his ability to adapt to the limitations imposed by his illness.*

Two behaviors are involved here: *identifies* and *analyzes*. A student may indeed identify phenomena but not be able to analyze them in relation to their influence on the patient's adaptive response. Actually, if the behavioral objective stated the one behavior, *analyze*, it would be sufficient because identification of phenomena is an integral part of the analytic process.

Exclusion of Methodology in Statement

Another pitfall for developers of behavioral objectives is the tendency to include methodology in the statement of the objective. This practice places a severe limitation on the learner as well as the evaluator, for it states that there is only one way the student can learn a particular behavior and it permits the evaluator to assess that student's competency only in terms of the method specified. For example, the following behavioral objective includes a methodology restriction:

The nursing student demonstrates collaborative skills through maintenance of effective interpersonal interactions.

This behavior as stated suggests that only one dimension of collaborative skill is emphasized: maintaining effective interpersonal interactions. Furthermore, the evaluator's assessment is restricted to competence in collaborative skills according to this one criterion. It ignores many other criteria, such as the learner's assessment of the problem under discussion; problem-solving ability; knowledge of nursing's particular contribution to the solution of the problem.

Another method may be injected into a statement of a behavioral objective. This method is the instructional procedure used to help the student attain the behavior. The following illustration includes a methodology, suggesting that a student's learning can be attained and validated only in terms of one procedure.

The nursing student develops through group discussion an awareness of the interrelationship between one's values and one's response to individuals with diverse life styles.

This objective suggests that this awareness is developed only in group discussions. Also, evaluation of the behavior must validate that learning occurred in group discussion. This approach is most unrealistic, for it is well known that individuals have many sources of learning and the student could have achieved this awareness through other life experiences.

A good guideline to remember when writing behavioral objectives is: when you find yourself ready to use words such as *through* or *by,* stop— because you are involving yourself with methodology.

Statements Rather Than a List of Topics

Occasionally one sees a list of topics representing theories, concepts, laws, or generalizations identified as the list of objectives for a particular educational experience. Previous discussions about behavioral objectives should indicate why such a list could not meet criteria for objectives. Objectives refer to actions expected of the learner. The topics, which in reality are content, suggest no action on the part of the learner. They offer no direction for program planning and certainly are impossible to evaluate.

What would the following list for a unit of a course mean?

Concept of stress
Adaptation process
Health-disease continuum
Nursing process

This list tells the reader only that these topics are included in the unit. There is no clue as to the depth to which they are to be explored nor to the focus of the exploration. Certainly, one has no idea what the learner is expected to do about these topics and therefore they cannot be evaluated. Thus, a list of topics shows the content area; it is not an objective.

ANALYSIS OF A BEHAVIORAL OBJECTIVE

Behavioral objectives are to be used by educators and students. Too often the development of behavioral objectives becomes an end in itself. After one faculty group had worked for some time in developing objectives for a course and reached a consensus on the objectives, one faculty member said, "Now that we have the objectives done, let's put them away and get down to identifying the content." How often this same behavior occurs! It would seem that some faculty may know how to write behaviors but they do not know what to do with them once they are developed.

Behavioral objectives tell much. The Behavioral Objective Analysis Direction Model (Fig. 3-1) provides an approach for using general behavioral objectives as a guide in all parts of the educational endeavor. This model states that behavioral objectives give direction to:

1. The behavior called for.
2. The content required.

Behavioral objectives provide clues to:

1. The method best suited to meet the objective. (Method is designated as the teaching activity of the teacher.)
2. The type of learning experience which enables the learner to accomplish the behavior desired in the objective. (Learning activity is designated as the activity in which the learner is involved.)
3. Methods and criteria for evaluation of the attainment of the objective.

It is in these three areas of method, learning experience, and evaluation that the opportunity for creativity and individualization of learning experi-

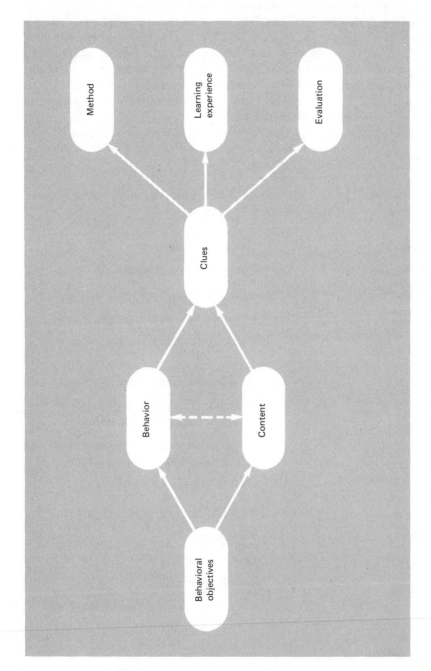

Figure 3-1. Behavioral Objective Analysis Direction Model.

ence occurs. The nature of the behavior and the content suggest possible approaches in these areas. We might use as an example a behavior that is a psychomotor skill. In this case methodology and learning experience must include a practice component, and evaluation must be through observation. However, these are not the only possible ways to follow through on this behavior, and an assortment of approaches developed in response to the clues provided by the behavior and content serve to provide variety in teaching, learning, and evaluation.

Earlier in this chapter, a general behavioral objective was presented. The analysis of that objective according to the Behavioral Objective Analysis Direction Model (Fig. 3-1) follows.

OBJECTIVE: The nursing student distinguishes the differences between male and female patterns of communication.

1. Behavior   Distinguish differences

2. Content   Communication process

                                            • Elements: message, sender, receiver

                                            • Means: verbal, nonverbal, graphic

Factors influencing the process

Differences in anatomical structure of male and female vocal apparatus

Influence of anatomical structure on verbal means of communication

Social and cultural influences on male and female communication patterns

CLUES

1. Method   Bibliography

Questioning

Group discussion

Visual aids—models, simulations, etc.

Audiovisual aids—films, slides, tapes, records

Supervised clinical practice

<table>
<tr><td></td><td>

CLUES *(cont.)*
</td></tr>
</table>

	CLUES *(cont.)*
2. Learning activity	Reading from selections on bibliography
	Listening to tapes, records
	Written paper
	Process recording
	Role playing
	Comparative study of male and female patient communication
	Oral presentation to peers
3. Evaluation	Clinical conference
	• Describe communication differences between male and female patients as each discussed some aspect of his or her care
	Written assignment
	• Describe differences in male and female communication as portrayed on slide tape in which a man and a woman read Rod McKuen's poem, "Knowing When to Leave"
	Library reference
	• Paper showing differences as noted by authorities
	Process recording of a male and female patient interaction analyzed for data, interpretation, and implications.

This analysis is not intended to be comprehensive, but it does illustrate the potential for making the behavioral objective operational. Analyses of the behavioral objectives suggest content relevant for the educational experience. Identification of a variety of methods and learning activities enables faculty and students to use paths toward attaining the objective that meet the needs of particular students and learning situations. Various approaches to evaluation will increase the data base concerning a student's competency or will individualize the evaluation so that it is specific for a given learner and/or situation need.

Once identified from all behavioral objectives designated for a particular educational experience, the content can then be organized in whatever logical fashion the faculty deems appropriate. Methodology and learning experiences are then selected as indicated in the analysis. The important point is that all parts of the educational experience are related to behaviors specified as desired outcomes.

MASTERY OF LEARNING CONCEPT APPLIED TO BEHAVIORAL OBJECTIVES

One question often raised by program developers relative to behavioral objectives is: for whom should behavioral objectives be designed—the average student, the top student, or the below-average student? The answer the teacher selects has much to do with his or her attitude toward and beliefs about the teaching-learning process and expectations of the learner's performance. If the expectations predicate that a certain percentage of students will succeed, another percentage will fail, and another percentage will partially meet the objectives, the teacher's academic goals have been formalized at least in attitude and the results will be consistent with these expectations. Indeed, a self-fulfilling prophesy has been created.

Bloom, Hastings, and Madaus (1965) in a chapter *Learning For Mastery*, address this issue and state, "Given sufficient time (and appropriate types of help), 95 percent of students (the top 5 percent plus the next 90 percent) can learn a subject up to a high level of mastery."[16] This conclusion is based on their studies of aptitude distributions, which indicate the following three groupings of students:

1. At the top of the distribution is 1 to 5 percent with a special talent for the subject and an ability to learn it quickly and with greater fluency than other students.
2. At the other extreme is less than 5 percent with special disability for a particular learning, e.g., a person who thinks in concrete forms would have difficulty with abstract concepts in nursing.
3. In between is 90 percent where aptitudes are predictive of rate of learning rather than the level (or complexity) of learning.

The mastery of learning concept does not say that 95 percent of the students *will achieve* mastery. It says only that they have the *potential*. Five variables are relevant to this concept and may be used effectively in our formative evaluation protocols. The five variables are:

1. Aptitude for a particular type of learning, which refers to the amount of time required by the learner to attain mastery of a learning task.

2. Quality of instruction, which refers to the degree to which the presentation, explanation, and ordering of elements of the task to be learned approach optimum for a given learner.
3. Ability to understand instruction, which refers to the learner's understanding of the nature of the task to be learned and the procedure to be followed in the learning of the task.
4. Perseverance, which refers to the time the learner is willing to put into learning.
5. Time allowed for learning, which is the key to the concept of aptitude.

Should we then say that 95 percent of the learners can master a particular behavioral objective, providing a strategy for mastery of learning is developed that considers individual differences among learners and accommodates the teaching-learning process to these differences? The teacher who enters a learning situation with such a goal in mind will be ready to diagnose student needs and provide support services and teaching strategies based on the diagnosis. The teaching-learning situation then tends to become a facilitating experience for all students, rather than a satisfying one for some.

As Bloom et al. suggest, a common practice in education programs is a misuse of the statistical theory, which works against the mastery of learning approach. The normal curve, which predicates that a certain percent of students will master a learning task, an equal number will fail, and the rest will fall in a rank on a scale, is based on the notion of chance in random activity. In nursing, learners do not represent a random sample; they are a highly selective group of individuals. Since our educational endeavors for this highly selective group is purposeful activity, the results of achievement should show a skewed curve. Bloom et al. point out the fallacy in using a normal curve to depict academic competency, stating: "In fact, we may even insist that our educational efforts have been unsuccessful to the extent to which our distribution of achievement approximates the normal distribution."[17]

The critical issue is not for what type of student the behavioral objectives should be developed, but rather what mastery of learning strategies should be instituted as the objectives become operational so that, except for the possible few who may have a special disability for that type of behavior, all students may succeed.

SUMMARY

Although there are several prescriptions for writing behavioral objectives, they usually can be classified into two categories, specific and general. Specific behavioral objectives include:

1. Description of the learner.
2. Description of the type of behavior expected.
3. Description of the conditions under which the learner demonstrates competence.
4. A statement of an acceptable standard of performance.

General behavioral objectives include the first two components, although the second component is often stated in two elements, behavior and content.

The intended use for the behavioral objective is the criterion used to assess the suitability of each type of objective rather than some concept of inherent worth.

Since behavioral objectives serve primarily as a means of communication for all parties involved in the educational endeavor, they must be written clearly and explicitly. Behavioral terms imply action, and the actions stated must be appropriate to the situation and must be measurable.

Behavioral objectives are to be used by program planners as well as by actual participants in the teaching-learning situation. They must be analyzed in terms of behavior, content, method, learning experience, and evaluation. The result of this analysis is then synthesized into the program of instruction.

Expectations of a student's ability to meet the behavioral objective greatly influence his/her attitude and that of the teacher as they come together for the educational experience. Recognition that at least 95 percent of the learners may attain the objective challenges the teacher to diagnose learning needs and to develop mastery of learning strategies.

REFERENCES

1. Kibler, R. J., Barker, L. L., & Miles, D. T. Behavioral Objectives and Instruction. Boston: Allyn & Bacon, 1970, p. 20.
2. Tanner, D. Using Behavioral Objectives in the Classroom. New York: Macmillan, 1972, p. 28.
3. Skinner B. F. The Technology of Teaching. New York: Appleton-Century-Crofts, 1968, p. 21.
4. Tanner D. *op cit*, p. 29.
5. Dewey J. Democracy and Education. New York: Macmillan, 1961, p. 340.
6. Whitehead A. N. The Aims of Education. New York: Macmillan, 1958 (Free Press), pp. 1, 2.
7. *Idem.* p. 3.
8. Boulding K. E. The Image. Ann Arbor, Mich.: University of Michigan, 1961, p. 14.
9. *Idem.* p. 17.
10. Tyler R. W. Basic Principles of Curriculum and Instruction. Chicago: University of Chicago, 1950, p. 28.
11. *Idem.* p. 37.
12. Bloom B. S., Englehart M. D., Furst E. J., Hill W. H., & Krathwohl D. R.

Taxonomy of Educational Objectives: Handbook I, Cognitive Domain. New York: David McKay, 1965, pp. 35-36.
13. Tanner D. *op cit.* p. 28.
14. Kibler R. J., Barker L. L., & Miles D. T. *op cit.* p. 20.
15. *Idem.* p. 321.
16. Bloom B. S., Hastings J. T., & Madaus G. F. Handbook on Formative and Summative Evaluation of Student Learning. New York: McGraw-Hill, 1971, p. 46.
17. *Idem.* p. 45.

RECOMMENDED READINGS

Bernabe R. & Leles S. Behavioral Objectives in Curriculum and Evaluation. Dubuque, Iowa: Kendall/Hunt, 1970.
Bigge M. Learning Theories for Teachers. New York: Harper and Row, 1964.
Block J.H. (ed). Mastery Learning: Theory and Practice. New York: Holt, Rinehart and Winston, 1971.
Conley V.C. Curriculum and Instruction in Nursing. Boston: Little, Brown, 1973.
Fivars, G. & Gosnell D. Nursing Evaluation: The Problem and the Process. New York: Macmillan, 1966.
Mager R. Preparing Educational Objectives. Palo Alto. Fearon: 1962.

4 Use of Taxonomy in Developing Behavioral Objectives for Nursing

A behavioral objective is not an isolate. It is part of a total phenomenon; as such it is related to all other behavioral objectives salient to that phenomenon. The boundaries of the phenomenon are circumscribed by some predetermined overall framework. In program planning this means that some system of ordering behavioral objectives must be utilized to provide for their interrelationship and for their expression in terms of developmental progress goals.

The system selected must answer nursing's concern for identification of levels of behavior that signify development within an educational program or relevancy to the needs of a particular group of learners. It must help program developers to identify specific behaviors that can be measured. Too often one finds such terms as *basic* knowledge, *increased* knowledge, and *greater* knowledge in statements of objectives. These adjectives, however, cannot be measured since they are not on a continuum within some acceptable framework. What is basic? Increased from what? Greater than what?

HOLISTIC NATURE OF MAN'S BEHAVIOR

Any system or approach to ordering behaviors according to a particular classification falls short in its ability to describe the totality of man's behavioral responses. Man is a thinking, feeling, acting, social being who responds as a total organism to stimuli from the environment. In some instances the components of man's behavior respond in harmony; at other times there is disunity among the components, with one or more predominating at any one time. Unity of response is wisdom, a goal toward which all learners should be directed. However, as the complexity of life interfaces with the complexity of human behavior, man finds that the search for wisdom is a life-long process.

Failure to recognize the imbalance between components of a person's behavioral response leads to unrealistic expectations and inappropriate actions. In the health field how often have we predicated our actions on the assumption that one's rational nature predominates, and thus ignored the role of custom, habit, motivation, and perception in determining how an individual will respond to our therapeutic regimens or health teaching.

Because the individual's behavioral responses to stimuli are holistic, program planners must recognize that the behavioral objectives of programs or any unit of teaching really represent multiple behaviors. This issue will be discussed in more detail later, but as the teacher develops programs and prepares for their evaluation, there must be an acknowledgment of the multidimensional character of one's behavior.

A TAXONOMY APPROACH

A system for ordering behaviors within the context of development—one which is being stressed by educators—is the taxonomy of educational objectives developed by Bloom, Krathwohl, and their associates. The reader is referred to two publications: Bloom (ed.) (1956): *Taxonomy of Educational Objectives, Handbook I: Cognitive Domain,* and David Krathwohl et al. (1964): *Taxonomy of Educational Objectives, Handbook II: Affective Domain.* These sources provide specific information relative to the theoretical basis for taxonomies, the process by which they were developed, and their application in educational programs. Some general areas for discussion should be mentioned as a basis for using the taxonomies in nursing educational endeavors.

Concept of Taxonomy

A taxonomy is a classification system. Bloom et al. (1956) developed such a system for educational goals; they agreed that the taxonomy should be an educational-logical-psychological classification system.[1]

> *Educational:* boundaries between categories to be closely related to distinctions teachers make in planning curricula and choosing learning experiences.

Logical: terms to be defined as precisely as possible and used consistently.

Psychological: concepts to be consistent with relevant and accepted psychological principles and theories.

Taxonomy then specifies the desired outcomes of an instructional endeavor. Krathwohl et al. (1964) observe that the meaning of educational objectives could be enhanced by using a taxonomy in which an objective is placed within a large overall scheme or matrix. They state, "Here it is hoped that placing the objective within the classification scheme would locate it on a continuum and thus serve to indicate what is intended as well as what is NOT intended."[2]

Rationale For Taxonomic System

The critical dimension of a taxonomic system, like the behavioral objectives themselves, is its potential for facilitating communication in matters of education to all concerned. There is a need for standardized terminology that is applicable to human behavioral responses which educators seek to evaluate. Abstract terms to describe these responses negate the possibility of evaluation.

Krathwohl et al. identify four values of a taxonomy to which he and his associates subscribed.[3]

1. The actual sharing in the process of classifying educational objectives would help members of the group clarify and tighten the language of educational objectives.
2. The classification scheme would provide a convenient system for describing and ordering test items, examination techniques, and evaluation instruments.
3. The scheme provides a means of studying and comparing educational programs.
4. Principles of classifying educational outcomes could reveal a real order among outcomes.

Taxonomy has a direct bearing on nursing programs as it helps nurse teachers assure ample high-quality objectives. Perusal of many examinations or other evaluative procedures supports the contention that recall of information is emphasized in education. Nurses *use* information, and it is their ability to use information in a variety of problem situations that should be evaluated. Likewise, in the affective domain, little if any attention is directed toward evaluating the valuing process and the internalization of values. As members of a helping profession nurses cannot remain in a state of awareness, the lowest level of affective behavior, relative to the worth and dignity of each human being. They must value each human being and internalize their values so that their behavior lends credence to their stated values. This means that higher affective behaviors must be emphasized in the nursing program.

A faculty or group using a taxonomy, then, must select methodology, learning experiences, and evaluation procedures related to the level of behavior deemed relevant to a particular group of learners. This level is selected from the range on the continuum of the taxonomy. Tanner (1972) sees the taxonomy system as "designed to classify the intended behaviors of students as a result of participating in some set of instructional experiences, and to be used in obtaining evidence on the extent to which such behaviors are manifest."[4]

Domains of Instructional Objectives

Learning behavior is manifested in three ways: (a) cognitive, the intellectual ability; (b) affective, the states of feeling, valuing; and (c) psychomotor, the manipulative and motor skills.

As described earlier in this chapter, most behavior that arises from learning is a composite of all three manifestations; yet educators have found it most useful to classify instructional objectives into the three domains: cognitive, affective, and psychomotor. Kibler, Barker, and Miles (1970) suggest three reasons for this method of classifying objectives:[5]

1. To avoid concentrating on one or two categories to the exclusion of others.
2. To make sure that instruction is provided for prerequisite objectives before attempting to teach more complex ones.
3. To assure that appropriate instruments are employed to evaluate desired objectives.

Bloom, Krathwohl, et al. noted the interdependence of these three domains in behavior as they developed the taxonomies, but they supported their decision for a separate taxonomy for the cognitive and the affective domains with the fact that teachers and curriculum workers do differentiate between problem-solving and attitudes as well as among acting, thinking, and feeling. Recognizing that any classification scheme that attempts to order phenomena does some injustice to them, as observed in practice, Krathwohl et al. feel that the "value of these attempts to abstract and classify is in their greater powers for organizing and controlling the phenomena. We believe the value of the present system of classification is likely to be in the greater precision with which objectives are likely to be stated, in the increased communicability of the objectives, and in the extent to which evaluation evidence will become available to appropriate student progress toward the objectives."[6]

Each of these domains represents a broad classification of human behavior and each is amenable to classification within its parameters on a progressive developmental continuum. Each category of behavior builds upon the skills identified in the category below it.

The identification of a specific behavioral objective within one of the behavioral domains is a professional judgment of program planners and is generally based on the decision to measure a particular skill. One has to realize, however, that these judgments do reflect the values of the planners, and care must be taken to assure that the domain selected is the proper one for a particular learning experience. Arbitrary decisions as to the classification of behavioral objectives could lead not only to emphasis on unimportant aspects of the situation, but also to emphases that are not consistent with the developmental needs of the learner.

We are what we learn. If analysis of a health problem involves only cognition of the biophysical component and ignores the nursing student's search for values as they relate to the solution of a problem, then much harm has been done to the learner. The input of self relative to feelings, beliefs, values, and attitudes must also be explored in problem-solving situations. Tanner stresses that developers of taxonomies of instructional objectives must recognize the continuity and interdependence of the three domains as he reminds the reader, ". . . it should be stressed that although the term domain implies a separation of spheres of activity, in effective learning these spheres are marked, not by separation and isolation, but by continuity and interdependence."[7] He further suggests that it would be useful for teachers and curriculum workers to examine these domains separately with a view toward:[8]

1. Developing teaching-learning strategies and evaluative measures that are more fully representative of the broad spectrum of cognitive goals that are attainable.
2. Developing teaching-learning strategies that are representative of affective goals relevant to the curriculum.
3. Developing needed interrelationships between cognitive and affective goals in the teaching-learning process and in the evaluation of achievement.

Within a nursing program Tanner's list should be expanded to include:

4. Developing teaching-learning strategies that are representative of the psychomotor competencies relevant to the practice of nursing.

Tanner's third item should be changed to state: developing needed inter-relationships among cognitive, affective, and psychomotor goals in the teaching-learning process and in the evaluation of achievement.

COGNITIVE DOMAIN

Examination of the curriculum and the evaluation strategies of many nursing programs would support findings by Bloom et al. that most educational objectives lie in the cognitive domain. The objectives range from simple recall to the complex processes of synthesis and validation through external and internal criteria. The principle of complexity is the basic one used in ordering intellectual skills in the taxonomy of the cognitive domain. Al-though this principle implies that cognitive learning occurs in a sequential pattern—from simple to complex behaviors—Tanner suggests that "this premise may be more of a logical ordering of cognitive behaviors rather than a truly valid explanation of a sequential development of various levels of cognitive behaviors."[9] Indeed, it is important not to place a value connota-tion on this hierarchy with the value increasing as the behaviors become more complex. The critical determinant is the appropriateness of the level of behavior to the nature of the problem to be solved or the skill to be acquired.

A condensed version of the *Taxonomy of the Cognitive Domain,* as de-veloped by Bloom et al., follows. Included is a brief description of the meaning of the terms and an illustration of a behavioral objective for each level. (The term *nursing student* used in the behavioral objectives refers to any nursing learner, whether engaged in a formal educational, a staff de-velopment, or a continuing education program.) It is suggested that before the taxonomy is used as a conceptual framework for developing cognitive behaviors, the original source should be consulted so as to maintain the integrity of the taxonomy as it is translated into a program.

The value of using a framework such as this taxonomy is that terms have meanings that facilitate communication. It is important, however, that the meaning of the terms, as designated by the developers, be adhered to. For instance, when the term *evaluation* is used in the taxonomy, it has a very special meaning, representing the high order of intellectual skill typified in the research process. In nursing one use of the term *evaluation* is in refer-ence to the final step in the nursing process. Evaluation in this context is one step in the problem-solving process in which a given set of data is used to determine results. Throughout the interpretations of each step in the taxonomy, one term appears regularly—the word *communication.* As one applies each step to the field of nursing, which is characterized by practice, interpretation of the term *communication* must be broadened to include actions in practice as well as the usual forms of written and oral communica-tion found in most general educational programs.

CONDENSED VERSION OF TAXONOMY OF COGNITIVE DOMAIN OF EDUCATIONAL OBJECTIVES*

Knowledge (Information)

1.00 *Knowledge*
Recall of specifics, universals, the recall of methods, processes, or the recall of a pattern, structure, or setting.

  1.10 *Knowledge of Specific*
Recall of specific and isolated bits of information, with emphasis on symbols with concrete referents.

    1.11 *Knowledge of Terminology*
Knowledge of the referents for specific symbols (verbal and nonverbal).

    Objective

    The nursing student defines the term *adaptation*.

    1.12 *Knowledge of Specific Facts*
Knowledge of dates, events, persons, places, source of information, properties, and phenomena.

    Objective

    The nursing student names the four chambers of the heart.

  1.20 *Knowledge of Ways and Means of Dealing with Specifics*
Recall of ways of organizing, studying, judging, and criticizing—chiefly in passive awareness of material rather than ability to use it.

    1.21 *Knowledge of Conventions*
Knowledge of characteristic ways of treating and presenting ideas and phenomena.

    Objective

    The nursing student identifies three ways by which nurses provide for the safety of the patient in a hospital setting.

    1.22 *Knowledge of Trends and Sequences*
Knowledge of the processes, directions, and movements of phenomena with respect to time.

---

*This condensed version is presented with permission of publisher, David McKay from Bloom, B.S. (ed.), Engelhart, M.D., Furst, E.J., Hill, W.H., and Krathwohl, D.R. *Taxonomy of Educational Objectives:* Handbook I, Cognitive Domain. New York:David McKay, 1956.

Objective

The nursing student identifies four trends in society that may influence the direction of the nursing profession in the future.

1.23 *Knowledge of Classifications and Categories*
Knowledge of the classes, sets, divisions, and arrangements regarded as fundamental for a given subject field, purpose, argument, or problem.

Objective

The nursing student names the classification of needs according to Maslow's hierarchy of human needs.

1.24 *Knowledge of Criteria*
Knowledge of the criteria by which facts, principles, opinions, and conducts are tested or judged.

Objective

The nursing student lists criteria to be used in assessing the effectiveness of an interview with a patient.

1.25 *Knowledge of Methodology*
Knowledge of methods of inquiry, techniques, and procedures employed in a particular subject field as well as those employed in investigating particular problems and phenomena.

Objective

The nursing student lists methods of data collection appropriate to assessing health needs of an individual.

1.30 *Knowledge of the Universals and Abstractions in a Field*
Recall of knowledge of the major ideas, schemes, and patterns by which phenomena and ideas are organized, such as theories and generalizations used in explaining phenomena and in solving problems.

1.31 *Knowledge of Principles and Generalizations*
Knowledge of particular abstractions that summarize observations of phenomena, i.e., explain, predict, describe, or determine most appropriate action.

Objective

The nursing student lists the scientific principles relevant to proper use of the sphygmomanometer in reading blood pressure.

1.32   *Knowledge of Theories and Structures*
Knowledge of the body principles and generalizations, together
with their interrelations, present a clear, rounded, and systematic
view of a complex phenomenon, problem, or field.

Objective

The nursing student lists three theories of human behavior that
may be used to interpret one's behavior in a stress situation.

Comprehension

2.00   *Comprehension*
The first level of intellectual skills relevant to understanding. At this
level the learner grasps the meaning of the communicated message
sufficiently well to use it in relating to other material or in solving a
problem without necessarily recognizing its fullest implication.

2.10   *Translation*
The expression of the communication in another language, into
other terms, or into another form of communication.

Objective

The nursing student gives an illustration of a nonverbal behavior
that impedes effective communication between the nurse and the
client.

2.20   *Interpretation*
The explanation or summary of a communication involving a rear-
rangement or a new perspective of the material.

Objective

The nursing student explains the aging process according to Erikson's theory of growth and development.

2.30   *Extrapolation*
The extension of trends or tendencies beyond given data and findings of the document to determine implications, consequences,
corollaries, effects, etc., which are in accordance with conditions as
literally described in the original communication.

Objective

The nursing student predicts the consequences of a therapeutic
nursing action from data collected about patients' health needs.

Application

3.00 *Application*
The intellectual skill referring to *use* of knowledge. It is the use of abstractions, such as ideas, principles, or theories in concrete situations.

Objective

The nursing student uses the nursing process in the care of individuals and groups within the usual health care settings.

Analysis

4.00 *Analysis*
Emphasis on the breakdown of material into its own constituent parts and detection of the relationship of parts and of the way they are organized. Deals with content and form of material, i.e., analysis of *meaning*. Uses resources outside of data at hand.

4.10 *Analysis of Elements*
Identification of elements of a communication, the overt and covert elements, differentiating nature of the statements such as facts, value, intent.

Objective

The nursing student identifies the measures used in meeting the survival needs of the patient in cardiac crisis.

4.20 *Analysis of Relationships*
The connections and interactions between elements and parts of a communication to include relationships between different kinds of evidence, consisting of part to part, element to element, relevance of elements or parts to central idea or thesis in the communication.

Objective

The nursing student contrasts the adaptive needs of the patient in a temporary acute illness with those of a patient with a progressive illness.

4.30 *Analysis of Organization Principles*
The organization, systematic arrangement and structure which hold a communication together.

Objective

The nursing student detects the form and pattern of a health team operation in a health care setting.

Synthesis

5.00 *Synthesis*
The putting together of elements and parts so as to form a whole, a pattern or structure not clearly there before.

5.10 *Production of a Unique Communication*
The development of a communication reflecting the student's perspective about some ideas, attitudes, etc.

Objective

The nursing student writes an essay depicting a position relative to the expanded care responsibilities of the nurse.

5.20 *Production of a Plan or Proposed Set of Operations*
The development of a plan of work or proposal of a plan of operations.

Objective

The nursing student proposes a plan for optimizing the use of the pediatric nurse clinician in a community setting.

5.30 *Derivation of a Set of Abstract Relations*
The development of a scheme for classifying or explaining certain data or phenomena or the deduction of propositions and relations from a set of basic propositions or symbolic representations.

Objective

The nursing student formulates a theoretical framework of nursing applicable to the health care of a family that resides in an inner city environment.

Evaluation

6.00 *Evaluation*
Judgments about value for the purpose of ideas, works, solutions, methods, materials, etc. Qualitative and quantitative judgments about extent to which material and methods satisfy criteria, which are either determined by the student or given to him.

6.10   *Judgments in Terms of Internal Evidence*
The evaluation of a communication or situation from such evidence as logical accuracy, consistency, and other internal criteria.

Objective

The nursing student validates own research study in terms of internal criteria which include clarity, accuracy, validity, reliability, precision of statements, and logic of conclusions from data and appropriate documentation.

6.20   *Judgments in Terms of External Criteria*
The evaluation of a communication or situation with reference to selected criteria as comparing a work against the highest known standards in its field.

Objective

The nursing student validates own research study in relation to valid and reliable studies in related areas.

The taxonomy presented here identifies a hierarchy of intellectual behaviors. Kibler et al. identify behaviors from the second level (comprehension) upward as intellectual skills and abilities. Vargar (1972), however, proposes another classification in Bloom's taxonomy[10]:

Knowledge   ⎫
Comprehension ⎬   understanding
Application   ⎬   concept formation
Analysis   ⎭

Synthesis   ⎫   creativity
Evaluation   ⎭

In this concept, understanding is viewed within the realm of problem-solving and relates to the ability to respond correctly to a new situation by using the correct rules. Concept formation, the ability to understand the meaning of a word when it is used, is the critical form of understanding for communication.[11] Creativity is viewed as the unique product of the learner, which meets criteria implicit in the objective.

The taxonomy does provide a continuum expressed as progressive development that can be useful to nurse teachers. The emphasis on higher intellectual skills should characterize the outcome of programs for professional students and practitioners. Planners of programs for the nonprofessional students and practitioners should select intellectual skills at a lower level on the taxonomy to be achieved by learners in these groups.

AFFECTIVE DOMAIN

Few will challenge the concept of behavioral objective development for the cognitive or psychomotor domains of learning, but there is less consensus among program planners about the appropriateness of affective behavioral objectives. The affective domain relates to ethics, the standards or principles of moral actions; moral judgment, the reasoning compatible with standards of right behavior; value indicators such as attitudes, interests, beliefs, and goals; and values themselves. "It is that part of an individual through which the self is expressed; it is often the source of motivation for behavior. It is a sphere of learning with its own defined limits, yet it is closely related to and often interfaces with the other two domains of learning, the cognitive and the psychomotor domains."[12]

The existence of an affective domain of learning is acknowledged, yet it is not subjected to the same pedagogical actions as the other two domains. Krathwohl et al. warn us about the consequences of subjecting the affective domain to equitable education processes. Referring to the process as an "opening of Pandora's box," they state:

> It is in this 'box' that the most influential controls are to be found. The affective domain contains forces that determine the nature of an individual's life and ultimately the life of an entire people. To keep the 'box' closed is to deny the existence of the powerful motivational forces that shape the life of each of us. To look the other way is to avoid coming to terms with the real.[13]

The affective domain is a significant force in the practice of nursing, for it provides for the humanistic expression of the theories and skills which are germane to nursing. There are values which are the legitimate concern of nurse educators that must be taught to future practitioners as well as continually developed in current practitioners.

What values do we teach? The values specified in the Bill of Rights of our Constitution, which pertain to all our citizenry, are of concern to all nurses. More specifically the values inherent in our practice are enunciated in the Code for Nurses and underline the Standards of Nursing Practice proposed by our professional organization, the American Nurses Association. It is important to remember that the values which are addressed in the curriculum are those stated in the above three documents. Faculty are not accountable for values which students choose as relevant to their own personal life styles.

One cannot discuss values in nursing practice without a consideration of the impact of anthropology on a knowledge of norms, values, and behaviors. A pluralism of value systems now characterizes a society, particularly in the western world. Many of these pluralistic systems arise from the multiplicity of cultural groups residing within a society. As the "melting pot" theory is losing its significance, the acceptance of multivaried culture groups is becoming more prevalent. Since each group has its own value system and seeks to maintain it while bringing it into accord with the larger society, members of the health field are finding their practices taking on different meanings. Recognition that the concepts of health, illness, and sick role have particular meanings to different groups makes it essential to respect these diversities in the process of health care ministration. Nursing's methodology, nursing process, enables it to value more these diversities, but nurses are challenged not to bias their assessments or interventions on the basis of own value system.

When there is a marked difference in the cultural group, it is relatively easy for one to accommodate to the differences. It is when differences are subtle that one is most likely to miss cultural clues. Similarity in skin color among a group of individuals does not predicate similarity in values and behaviors. A group's life experiences as influenced by genetic and cultural roots, habitat location, customs, and systems of communication determine these values, which in turn direct its behavior.

If the affective domain is perceived as a legitimate and indispensable area of learning, then it is essential that affective behavioral objectives be identified for a particular learning experience. These behavioral objectives must then lend themselves to analysis in terms of behavior, content, method, learning experiences, and evaluation. It is true that educators are less than confident in their ability to operationalize affective behavioral objectives and to develop appropriate appraisal devices. Johnson (1973) sees the value question as a critical one in higher education and pleads for clarification of higher education's responsibility for value development. He states: "The student must cease to be the 'dependent variable' and begin to be the central developmental objective before which all other considerations pale in significance."[14]

Krathwohl et al. accepted the legitimacy of behavioral objectives in the affective realm and adopted the concept that affective behaviors could be developed when appropriate learning experiences were provided. Their search for an organizing principle that would enable them to devise a continuum of development led to the principle of internalization. This principle refers to "a process by which a given phenomenon or value passed from a level of bare awareness to a position of some power to guide or control the behavior of the person."[15] This process really refers to that inner growth of the individual by which is developed a value system which guides behavior in making choices for action.

Valuing Process

The principle of internalization selected by Krathwohl et al. in preparing the taxonomy of the affective domain is consistent with the ideas of the value theory proposed by Raths et al. They identify seven criteria for a value, *all* of which must be satisfied. They also indicate that the following criteria describe the process of valuing.[16]

1. Choosing freely
2. Choosing from among alternatives
3. Choosing after thoughtful consideration of the consequences of each alternative
4. Prizing and cherishing
5. Affirming publicly
6. Acting upon choices
7. Repeating, in some pattern of life

The process described involves considerable cognitive action, especially since a value must reflect a choice an individual has made. Thus the internalization process includes intellect and feeling, with the two closely intertwined at the upper level of the hierarchy. The critical factor in the internalization process is action consistent with a stated value. How often have we encountered the intellectualizer who espouses values verbally but fails to act consistently with them when called to do so! A nurse who professes to respect the worth and dignity of the individual but whose actions signify only "man with a life style compatible with the nurse's concept of *the right one*" has not internalized that value.

The hierarchy proposed by Krathwohl et al. reflects the seven criteria proposed by Raths et al., for both require that intellect and emotion blend. There are, however, some affective expressions that do not meet all seven criteria and thus cannot be considered values. Raths et al. see these as potential values and call them *value indicators* as long as they do not meet all seven criteria. These expressions include:[17]

1. Goals and purposes
2. Aspirations
3. Attitudes
4. Interests
5. Feelings
6. Beliefs and convictions
7. Activities
8. Worries, problems, obstacles

Raths, Harmin, and Simon (1966) provide the value development theory, the Nursing Code and Standards of Practice identify the values inherent in nursing practice, and Krathwohl et al. provide the affective domain taxonomy which enable the program planner to state affective behaviors according to a sequencing which leads to internalization. The first two levels of the taxonomy relate to value indicators. It is at the third level, valuing, that the choice is made and internalization begins.

Following is a condensed version of the *Taxonomy of the Affective Domain* as developed by Krathwohl et al. It includes a brief description of the meaning of terms and an illustration of a behavioral objective for each level.

CONDENSED VERSION OF TAXONOMY OF AFFECTIVE DOMAIN OF EDUCATIONAL OBJECTIVES*

Receiving

1.0 *Receiving* (Attending)
Sensitivity to the existence of a given condition, phenomenon, situation, or problem.

1.1 *Awareness*
Conscious recognition of the existence of a given condition, phenomenon, situation, or problem. Individual's attention is attracted to stimuli but there is no requirement to evaluate or verbalize.

Objective

The nursing student expresses an awareness of the need to involve the patient and family in developing a plan of care.

1.2 *Willingness to Receive*
A willingness to give attention to or note a phenomenon rather than to avoid it. Response is neutral and judgment is suspended.

Objective

The nursing student listens to the patient express concerns.

1.3 *Controlled or Selected Action*
Differentiation, selection, or discrimination among various aspects of a phenomenon. Involves differentiation of aspects of stimuli and/or attention to certain stimuli. Favored stimulus is selected and attended to.

*The condensed version is presented with permission of publisher, David McKay, from Krathwohl, D.R., Bloom, B.S., Masia, B.B. *Taxonomy of Educational Objectives*, Handbook II: Affective Domain. New York:David McKay, 1968.

Objective

The nursing student listens to comments made by nurses that suggest stereotypic views of various categories of people.

2.0 *Responding*
Reacting overtly to a stimulus or phenomenon, and doing something with or about them.

  2.1 *Acquiescence in Responding*
Complying with expectations, especially of those individuals in authority.

Objective

The nursing student reads the required references listed in the course bibliography.

  2.2 *Willingness to Respond*
Voluntary action in response to a given phenomenon reflecting a choice for the action.

Objective

The nursing student seeks opportunities for the mother of a sick child to participate in care.

  2.3 *Satisfaction in Response*
Enjoyment in acting on or responding to a given phenomenon. Emotional significance is now being attached to the stimulus.

Objective

The nursing student shares readily with peers experiences in interacting with patients and families.

Valuing

3.0 *Valuing*
A step in the internalization process signified by the attachment of worth or belief. Behavior is sufficiently consistent and stable to be characteristic of a belief or attitude.

  3.1 *Acceptance of a Value*
Belief in a phenomenon, behavior, object, etc., with reasonable certainty and sufficient internalization to be a controlling force. A willingness to be identified as one holding that belief.

Objective

The nursing student supports the rights of individuals to their own philosophies, moral codes, and life styles.

3.2 *Preference for a Value*

A willingness to pursue or seek out activities related to a phenomenon or belief that one has attached worth to and therefore is willing to be identified with.

Objective

The nursing student assumes responsibility for involving patients and their families in decisions of care that affect their lives.

3.3 *Commitment*

Belief with a high degree of certainty leading to conviction and involvement in the cause, principle, or doctrine. The individual is perceived as holding the value and motivated to act out the behavior.

Objective

The nursing student acts in an advocate role when patients' human rights are threatened in a patient care setting.

Organization

4.0 *Organization*

Development of values into an organized system after considering their interrelationships and establishing value priorities.

4.1 *Conceptualization of a Value*

The quality of abstraction or conceptualization is added to stability and consistency. Relationship between a value and the ones already held or new is involved.

Objective

The nursing student formulates judgments about nursing responsibilities relative to extraordinary means of maintaining life in a critically ill patient.

4.2 *Organization of a Value System*

Development of a complex of values, including disparate ones, into an ordered relationship that is both harmonious and internally consistent. Relationship of values is more likely to be described as a kind of dynamic equilibrium that is, in part, dependent upon portions of the environment relevant at any point in time.

Objective

The nursing student formulates a plan of action consistent with own values when confronted with decisions involving moral issues relevant to quality of life.

Characterization By a Value or Value Complex

5.0 *Characterization by a Value or Value Complex*
Internalization of a philosophy of life resulting from internalization of values; organization of an internally consistent system of values; and a consistent behavior pattern so that the individual is described in terms of his unique personal characteristics. The relationship between cognitive and affective processes is pronounced.

5.1 *Generalized Set*
Basic orientation that enables individual to reduce and order the complex world about him/her and to act consistently and effectively in it.

Objective

The nursing student judges health care problems in terms of issues, purposes, situations, and consequences rather than fixed dogmatic precepts, stereotypic ideas, and emotional wishful thinking.

5.2 *Characterization*
Internalization of a value system having as its object the whole of what is known, or knowable, with an internal consistency.

Objective

The nursing student develops a philosophy of life based on a personal and professional code of ethics that denotes his or her participation in improving the health and welfare of all members of society.

The taxonomy described here presents a hierarchy of value development toward the ultimate goal of self actualization. Individuals will be at different stages of the internalization process relative to different values at any point in time. Development is not a static process in which a value becomes permanently entrenched, but rather one that subjects the value to constant analysis and testing as the individual is called upon to make behavioral decisions in a world that is constantly changing.

PSYCHOMOTOR DOMAIN

A taxonomy for the psychomotor domain of learning has not been developed to the level of sophistication and utility that one finds for other domains, perhaps because in the literature there is less evidence of objectives written for this type of competency. Psychomotor skills, however, are significant in nursing practice and a taxonomy is needed to guide their development in an educational program.

The concept of psychomotor skills should be delineated sharply so that an organizing principle can be identified for the taxonomy. For this discussion, the psychomotor domain will be developed consistent with the definition offered by Dave (1970) and refers to "those behaviors which include muscular action and require neuromuscular coordination."[18]

Again the reader is reminded that human behavior is a holistic phenomenon, and all three domains are involved. Performing a psychomotor skill includes cognitive and affective behaviors. In Chapter 3 it was noted that acts of cognition and affection are inferred from psychomotor acts. A performance behavior involves the gestalt, whereas a psychomotor skill, as defined herein, involves neuromuscular coordination.

Educational literature contains several approaches to the classification of psychomotor behavior. Simpson proposed a scheme that includes the following five stages:[19]

1. Perception
2. Set
3. Guided response
4. Mechanism
5. Complex overt response

Kibler et al. developed a classification of behaviors that is not intended as a taxonomy per se. The behaviors involve:[20]

1. Gross body movements
2. Finely coordinated body movements
3. Nonverbal communication behaviors
4. Speech behaviors

Dave proposed a taxonomy that has considerable potential for nursing education. The organizing principle of his taxonomy is coordination. With suggested relevancy to nursing, this taxonomy is presented here as a possible approach. It does not have the authenticity of the other two taxonomies, but research should determine its validity and reliability. Five major steps are listed in the present taxonomy; perhaps refinement would suggest interim steps under each major heading.

Psychomotor Levels*

1.0 *Imitation*
When the learner is exposed to an observable action, he/she begins to make covert imitation of that action. Such covert behavior appears to be the starting point in the growth of psychomotor skill. This is then followed by overt performance of an act and capacity to repeat it. The performance, however, lacks neuromuscular coordination or control and hence is generally in a crude and imperfect form (i.e., impulse, overt repetition).

Interpretation

This behavior would be the learner's first experience following a demonstration by the nursing instructor or a viewing of a demonstration on a film or videotape.

Objective

The nursing student uses the sphygmomanometer to obtain a blood pressure reading on a patient.

2.0 *Manipulation*
Developing skill in following directions, performing selected actions, and fixing performance through necessary practice are emphasized. At this level, the learner is capable of performing an act according to instruction rather than only by observation, as in the case at the level of imitation (i.e., following directions).

Interpretation

At this stage the learner would be familiar with written nursing procedure and be able to use it as a guide in carrying out a skill.

Objective

The nursing student takes the patient's blood pressure reading, according to accepted procedure.

*By Dr. R.H. Dave, Head of Department of Curriculum and Evaluation, National Institute of Education, NIE Building, Nehraul Road, New Delhi.

3.0 *Precision*
Performance efficiency of a given act reaches a higher level of refinement. The learner performs the skill independent of a model or set of directions. Here accuracy, proportion, and exactness in performance become significant (i.e., reproduction, control, errors reduced to a minimum).

Interpretation

At this stage the learner is secure enough to carry out the skill independently with a high degree of accuracy.

Objective

The nursing student takes a patient's blood pressure reading accurately and in a manner consistent with scientific principles.

4.0 *Articulation*
Coordination of a series of acts is emphasized by establishing an appropriate sequence, achieving harmony or internal consistency among different acts (i.e., performance involves accuracy and control plus elements of speed and time).

Interpretation

This is the stage at which the learner blends all of the steps and variables bearing upon a skill. The skill is carried out smoothly within a reasonable time frame. Coordination is achieved.

Objective

The nursing student measures the patient's blood pressure competently, according to criteria of accuracy, smoothness, and reasonableness of time.

5.0 *Naturalization*
A high level of proficiency is required to perform a single act skillfully. The act is performed with the least expenditure of psychic energy. It is routinized to such an extent that it becomes an automatic and spontaneous response (i.e., performance becomes natural and smooth).

Interpretation

This is the stage at which the nursing learner shifts focus relative to psychomotor skill. The skill becomes a means to an end rather than an end in itself.

Objective

The nursing student integrates the taking of a patient's blood pressure reading into the total therapeutic plan for that patient.

As stated earlier, this scheme is presented here because it has potential for nursing education. Focus on the organizing principle of coordination does force the nursing teacher to concentrate on the psychomotor skill itself rather than on the total gestalt, especially during the early stages of development. Learning psychomotor skills is an egocentric process that absorbs the learner's attention until, as suggested here, Phase 5 (naturalization) is reached. The learner needs the assurance that hands, feet, or even the total body, will "work" in unison to give desired results, before the skill can be viewed in relation to the total phenomenon.

How many times in the process of teaching medicine administration have nursing instructors interrupted the student pouring medications with a question such as, "What are the toxic symptoms of the drug?" Emphasis in the learning experience is shifted from the skill to the content. How would a student driver, in his first experience driving a car on the highway, respond to a question such as, "What is the function of the spark plug in the engine?" Perhaps a taxonomy such as that suggested by Dave would make the skill a focal point of the learning experience and relegate content and value discussions to pre- and post-conferences until confidence in carrying out the psychomotor skill has been achieved.

TABLE 4.1

Behavioral Verbs Appropriate For Each Level of the Three Taxonomies

I. Cognitive
   C1.0 Information

define	name
identify	recall
list	recognize

   C2.0 Comprehension
      C2.1 Translation level

cite examples of	give in own words

      C2.2 Interpretation level

choose	discriminate
demonstrate use of	explain
describe	interpret
differentiate	select

C2.3 Extrapolation level

conclude	estimate
detect	infer
determine	predict
draw conclusions	

C3.0 Application

apply	generalize
develop	relate
employ	use

C4.0 Analysis

appraise	detect
compare	distinguish
contrast	evaluate
criticize	identify
deduce	

C5.0 Synthesis

classify	produce
design	reconstruct
develop	restructure
modify	synthesize
organize	systematize

C6.0 Evaluation

appraise	evaluate
assess	judge
critique	validate

II. Affective

A1.0 Receiving

acknowledges	shows awareness of
shares	

A2.0 Responding

acts willingly	practices
discusses willingly	responds
expresses satisfaction in	seeks opportunities
is willing to support	selects
listens to	shows interest

A3.0 Valuing

accepts	cooperates with
acclaims	helps
agrees	participates in
assists	respects
assumes responsibility	supports

A4.0 Organization of Values

argues	formulates a position
debates	is consistent
declares	takes a stand
defends	

(Continued)

    A5.0 Characterization by Value

              acts consistently   stands for
              is accountable

III. Psychomotor Behaviors According to Taxonomy

    P1.0 Imitation

              follows example of
              follows lead of

    P2.0 Manipulation

              , carries out according   follows procedure
                to procedure   practices

    P3.0 Precision

              demonstrates skill in using

    P4.0 Articulation

              carries out   uses
              is skillful in using

    P5.0 Naturalization

              is competent   carries out
              is skilled

SUMMARY

Man's behavior is a holistic process, as it responds to stimuli from the environment. This behavior is bounded by parameters of specific phenomena and is related to all other behaviors that occur at the same time. Program developers need a system for ordering behavioral objectives so as to provide for their interrelationships and expression in terms of directional progress goals.

A taxonomy of behavioral objectives, signifying a progressive development as determined by some organizing principle, provides a schema by which an objective can be placed on a continuum. Taxonomy facilitates communication among participants in the educational endeavor, clarifies the intended outcome, and promotes more acumen in evaluation.

Learning is expressed in three domains: cognitive, affective, and psychomotor. Although these three domains really are interdependent, development of a separate taxonomy for each is compatible with current teaching practices. It also assures that all three domains receive equitable emphasis in the program and guide participants in the selection of appropriate learning experiences as well as in the development of suitable evaluation strategies.

Bloom et al. developed a taxonomy of educational objectives for the cognitive domain using the concept of complexity as the organizing principle. Krathwohl et al. developed a taxonomy of educational objectives for the affective domain using the concept of internalization as the organizing principle. Both taxonomies are amenable to nursing education. A psychomotor taxonomy has not been formalized to the degree of sophistication found in the other two domains, but Dave's framework, based on the concept of coordination, points the way to a taxonomy directly applicable to nursing education.

REFERENCES

1. Bloom, B.S. (ed), Englehart M.D., Furst, E.J., Hill, W.H. & Krathwohl D.R. Taxonomy of Educational Objectives: Handbook I, Cognitive Domain. New York:David McKay, 1956, p. 6.
2. Krathwohl, D.R., Bloom, B.S., & Masia, B.B. Taxonomy of Educational Objectives: Handbook II, Affective Domain. New York:David McKay, 1964, p. 4.
3. *Idem.* p. 4.
4. Tanner, D. Using Behavioral Objectives in the Classroom. New York:Macmillan, 1972, p. 2.
5. Kibler, R.J., Barker, L.L., & Miles, D.T. Behavioral Objectives and Instruction. Boston:Allyn & Bacon, 1970, p. 44.
6. Krathwohl, D.R., Bloom, B.S., & Masia, B.B. *op. cit.*, p. 8.
7. Tanner, D. *op. cit.*, pp. 4-5.
8. *Idem.* p. 8
9. *Idem.* p. 21.
10. Vargas, J.S. Writing Worthwhile Behavioral Objectives. New York: Harper and Row, 1972, p. 105.
11. *Idem.* p. 98.
12. Reilly, D.E. Teaching and Evaluating the Affective Domain In Nursing Programs. Thorofare, N.J.: Charles B. Slack Inc., 1978, p. 32.
13. Krathwohl, D.R., Bloom, B.S., & Masia B.B. *op cit.*, p. 91.
14. Johnson, K.W. A Teacher's Influence: The Value Question in Higher Education. The Research Reporter 8:8, 1973.
15. Krathwohl, D.R., Bloom B.S., & Masia, B.B. *op. cit.*, p. 27.
16. Raths, L.E., Harmin, M., & Simon S.B. Values and Teaching. Columbus, Ohio: Merrill, 1966, pp. 28-30.
17. *Idem.* pp. 30-34.
18. Dave, R.H. Psychomotor Levels. In Developing and Writing Behavioral Objectives. Tucson, Arizona: Educational Innovators Press, 1970, p. 33.
19. Simpson, E.J. A Classification of Educational Objectives: Psychomotor Domain. Illinois Teachers of Home Economics 10:110, 1966.
20. Kibler, R.J., Barker, L.L., & Miles D.T. *op. cit.*, pp. 66-75.

RECOMMENDED READINGS

Allport, G. The Nature of Prejudice. Garden City, New York:Doubleday Anchor Books, 1958.

Bernabe, R. & Leles, S. Behavioral Objectives in Curriculum and Evaluation. Dubuque, Iowa:Kendall/Hunt, 1970.

Bidwell, C.M. & Froebe, D.J. Development of an Instrument for Evaluating Hospital Nursing Performance. J. Nurs. Admin., 1:10, 1971.

Bloom, B.S., Hastings, J.T., & Madaus, G.F. Handbook on Formative and Summative Evaluation of Student Learning. New York:McGraw-Hill, 1971.

Dichoff, J. & James, P. Beliefs and Values: Basis for Curriculum Design. Nurs. Res, 19:415, 1970.

Dressel, P.L. Values, Cognitive, and Affective: Editorial. J. Hyg. Educ., 92:400, 1971.

Englehardt, H.T., Jr. & Callahan, D. (eds). Knowledge, Value and Belief. Vol. 2. The Foundations of Ethics and its Relationship to Science. New York:Hastings Center, Institute of Society, Ethics and Life Sciences, 1977.

Englehardt, J.T. Jr. & Callahan, D. (eds). Morals, Science and Sociality Vol. 3. The Foundations of Ethics and its Relationship to Science. New York:The Hastings Center, Institute of Society, Ethics and Life Sciences, 1978.

Gardner, J.W. Morale. New York:W.W. Norton and Co. Inc., 1978.

Harmes, H.M. Behavioral Analysis of Learning Objectives. West Palm Beach, Florida:Harmes Assoc. 1969.

Illich, I. Medical Nemesis. New York:Random House, 1976.

Inlow, G.M. Values in Transition: A Handbook. New York:Wiley, 1972.

Kohlberg, L. From Is to Ought. In T. Mischele, (ed): Cognitive Development and Epistemology. New York:Academic Press, 1971.

Kohlberg, L. The Child as a Moral Philosopher. Psych. Today, 2:28, September 1968.

Kohlberg, L. The Cognitive-Developmental Approach to Moral Education. Humanist, 32:12-18. November/December 1972.

Moore, W. Jr. Against the Odds. San Francisco:Jossey-Bass, 1970.

Rogers, C. Freedom to Learn. Columbus, Ohio:Charles B. Merrill, 1969.

Schesbe, K.E. Beliefs and Values. New York:Holt Rinehart and Winston, 1970.

Shetland, M. The Responsibility of the Professional School for Preparing Nurses for Ethical, Moral, and Humanistic Practice. Nurs. For., 8:17, 1969.

Simon, S.B., Howe, L.W., & Kirschenbaum, H. Values Clarification. New York:Hart, 1972.

Spector, R. Cultural Diversity in Health and Illness. New York:Appleton-Century-Crofts, 1979.

Steele, S.M. & Harmon V.M. Values Clarification in Nursing. New York:Appleton-Century-Crofts, 1979.

Wales, C.E. Educational Systems Design. Eng. Educ., 62:844, 1969.

Wojcik, J. Muted Consent. West Lafayette, Indiana:Purdue Research Foundation, 1978.

5 Systematic Approach to the Development of Behavioral Objectives in a Nursing Program

As has been previously stated, a behavioral objective or a set of behavioral objectives does not exist in a vacuum, but is always part of a larger system. Within the larger system such objectives contribute to its viability and in turn derive vitality from it.

A systems approach to educational programs is not new to nursing. Following the medical model, nursing programs developed around body systems, and nursing care was taught as specifically related to each system. Modern systems theories directed nursing into a search for a systems model that is more representative of nursing practice. Chin (1961) refers to a conceptual model of practice when he states, "All practitioners have ways of thinking about and figuring out situations of change. These ways are embedded in the concepts with which they apprehend the dynamics of the client system they are working with, their relationship to it, and their process of helping with the change."[1]

It is not within the scope of this book to present conceptual models for nursing or for nursing education. This chapter, however, does demonstrate a systematic approach to the evolution of behavioral objectives within a nursing education program.

DEVELOPMENTAL MODEL

A system may be conceptualized as a phenomenon, a gestalt, composed of parts or elements, and as connected to each other so that interaction, interdependence, and integration occur. Boundaries of a particular system represent a closure around selected variables of the phenomenon, so that the energy exchange occurs primarily within the closure and little occurs between the system and its outside environs. Parts of the system may be referred to as subsystems, each with its own structure and function and a certain degree of autonomy. Each subsystem has its own goals and energy for self maintenance, growth, and self perpetuation. It is open and connected to other subsystems, and thus is susceptible to a disturbance in other parts of the subsystem.

Chin's developmental model is compatible with the concept of education as a force expediting the development of human potential. Chin characterizes the developmental model in the following manner:

> *By developmental models, we mean those bodies of thought that center around growth and directional change. Developmental models assume change; they assume that there are noticeable differences between the states of a system at different times; that the succession of these states implies the system is heading somewhere; and that there are orderly processes which explain how the system gets from its present state to where it is going.* [2]

In this model, one may refer to stages rather than to subsystems, but each stage can be identified and each meets the characteristics described for subsystems. With this model the learner's growth and development become critical variables, and behavioral objectives are expressed in terms of directional progress goals. Since the taxonomies, as described in previous chapters, are also predicated on the assumption that growth in each of the three domains (cognitive, affective, and psychomotor) is the main goal of educational endeavors, the taxonomies provide a methodology for the developmental model of behavioral objectives.

SYSTEM IN NURSING EDUCATION PROGRAMS

For our present purposes, it can be said that the system involves behavioral objectives of the program as well as all stages or subsystems of the program related to objectives. It is important to remind the reader, however, that the derivation of the program of behavioral objectives results from an exploration of seven areas; nature of man, societal trends and goals, professional issues and trends, nature of the learner, nature of the teaching-learning process, philosophy of the agency offering the program, and the theoretical construct of the nursing discipline.

The system of the program for the school of nursing would include subsystems of behavioral objectives, as shown in the Systems Model of Program Objectives (Fig. 5-1).

Program behavioral objectives are those a faculty and other participants in program planning determine as desirable outcomes. In some instances these

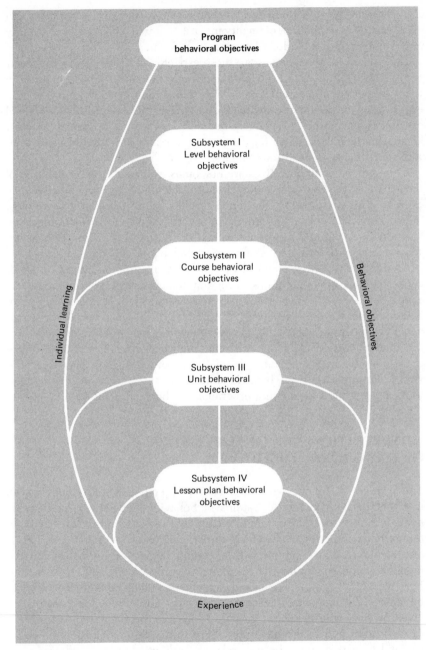

Figure 5-1. Systems Model of Program Behavior Objectives.

objectives are referred to as *terminal* objectives. The word *terminal,* however, carries a connotation of finality inconsistent with concepts of continuity in development and life-long learning.

Level behavioral objectives are those expected of a learner at a particular point in time in the program. The time dimension may be defined in terms of years in a program, completion of a certain group of courses or learning experiences, or period in which an individual has reached a designated level of competency. Since learning is perceived as a developmental process, levels should not occur at too frequent intervals; this would ensure that sufficient time is allowed for change.

Course behavioral objectives are outcomes expected at the conclusion of the course. If the course is divided into units, then behavioral objectives are expressed for each unit. If the nurse teacher uses individual lesson plans, then appropriate behavioral objectives are identified. Behavioral objectives for individual learning experiences may be chosen to flow from any of the subsystems or directly from the program behavioral objective (Fig. 5-1).

Modifications in the model will be made for continuing education or for in-service education programs. Program behavioral objectives would, of course, be the initial stage. Level behavioral objectives exist if the program is based within a developmental context identifiable in stages. Course behavioral objectives come into consideration if courses or unified blocks of learning are designed for the program. Inclusion of unit behavioral objectives depends on the organization of the program. Lesson plan and individual learning experience behavioral objectives are similar in development to these suggested for nursing programs in schools of nursing.

INTERRELATIONSHIP OF SUBSYSTEMS OF BEHAVIORAL OBJECTIVES

The Systems Model of Program Behavioral Objectives (Fig. 5-1) connotes an interrelationship among subsystems of behavioral objectives; yet, in too many instances each subsystem is treated as a separate entity. Each subsystem of behavioral objectives meets the criteria of a subsystem; each has its own structure and functions with a certain degree of autonomy and demonstrates the energy for self maintenance, growth, and self perpetuation. However, other criteria—open and connected to other subsystems—seem to be ignored by many nurse teachers, with autonomy of the subsystem being given primary consideration. If, within a system, all subsystems contribute to each other and to the totality of the system, then all subsystems of behavioral objectives must be interrelated. Individuals responsible for planning behavioral objectives at each level do not have complete autonomy; rather, they must be certain that their planning is consistent with that of other parts of the system.

Program development moves from general to specific; that is, program behavioral objectives are determined first. Then, using a developmental concept, level behavioral outcomes are defined. The number of levels depends on their definition as described by the planners. Last level and program behavioral objectives are the same; for example, behavioral objectives for the senior year of a baccalaureate program are the same as program behavioral objectives since it is assumed that the learner will meet criteria for the latter by the end of the program.

Planners determine the framework for courses within each level, and behavioral objectives for each course are written accordingly. If a level represents a considerable time span, such as a year in a nursing program, it must be remembered that the planners perceived that period of time as essential for most learners to achieve the competency described. Therefore, behavioral objectives for courses that terminate earlier would be at a lower developmental level. Single behaviors identified primarily with a course, such as skill in listening to a fetal heart, are defined according to the expectation of faculty involved and not limited by behavioral objectives at a given level.

Unit behavioral objectives are derived from course behavioral objectives, and lesson plan behavioral objectives are derived from unit behavioral objectives. Individual learning experience behavioral objectives vary in their source, arising from behavioral objectives for any part of the system.

The process of producing behavioral objectives within this system utilizes the Chin developmental model as a framework, and the taxonomies as the method for identifying behaviors in each stage of development.

INTERDOMAIN BEHAVIORS

Before demonstrating the process, more needs to be said about behavioral objectives as written for each subsystem. As stated previously, a behavior is multidimensional, often involves two or more domains of learning, and is a composite of a series of behaviors. The domain selected as the primary focus of the behavioral objective is a judgment made by the planners, but behaviors that comprise a behavioral objective may represent all domains. Therefore when behavioral objectives for any of the stages are written, they must include the composite of behaviors accepted as evidence of achievement of the objective. The behaviors also bring into sharp focus those methodologies and learning experiences relevant to the behavioral objective.

Following is a behavioral objective with its components for data analysis in the nursing process. It is at the level expected of a practitioner.*

*The 'C' before the behavior means cognitive domain and the 'A' means affective domain.

BEHAVIORAL OBJECTIVE

C4.2   The nursing practitioner deduces relevancies and interrelationships of patient data.

BEHAVIORS

C4.2   Interprets data in terms of scientific theories, concepts, and principles.

C4.2   Relates the patient's response to health or illness to his sociocultural background.

A3.3   Accepts responsibility for valid data interpretation, free from individual prejudices.

C4.2   Uses appropriate resources for clarifying ambiguities in data.

C4.1   Identifies resources of patient and/or family for managing health needs.

A3.3   Accepts rights of patients and families to their own philosophies, moral codes, and life styles when drawing conclusions from data.

C4.2   Distinguishes discrepancies between own data analysis and that identified for a typical situation.

C4.2   Identifies significant relationships among data.

C4.2   Draws conclusions from data relationships.

In the above example, the behavioral objective is identified within the cognitive domain at the analytic level, according to the taxonomy. Nine behaviors, representative of affective and cognitive domains, are described for this behavioral objective. In this illustration, the psychomotor domain is not relevant. The level ascribed to the behavioral objective would be expected of a senior professional student or a professional practitioner. Behaviors of the domain identified in the behavioral objective are generally expressed within the same level as the objective; although there may be reasons that lead faculty to expect students to reach a higher or lower level of competency in a particular behavior.

Not only may behaviors within a behavioral objective represent different domains of learning, but so, too, may the development of behavioral objectives, or behaviors listed under the objective, change in domain as they progress through the system. In the discussion of affective behaviors, it was noted that cognition is an important part of the valuing process. Thus in the development of values, behaviors may first be expressed in the affective domain, then in the cognitive domain, and once again in the affective domain. Using an affective behavior from the above example as an illustration, the development process in a nursing program with three levels would be:

Level I   A1.2   The nursing student expresses an awareness of the relationship between a nurse's prejudices and the ability to assess a patient's needs accurately.

Level II   C2.3   The nursing student makes inferences from the theory of prejudice about the impact of own prejudices on the ability to assess patients' needs.

Level III   A3.3   The nursing student accepts responsibility for valid data interpretation free from the influence of individual prejudices.

In some instances, the affective behavior development may move from cognitive to affective through several levels of affective. Using the previous example, the development would be:

Level I   C2.3   The nursing student makes inferences from the theory of prejudice about the impact of individual prejudices on the ability to assess patients' needs.

Level II   A3.3   The nursing student accepts responsibility for valid data interpretation free from the influence of individual prejudices.

Level III   A4.2   The nursing student formulates judgments as to the nurse practitioner's responsibility to have individual prejudices under control when making patient assessments.

The Level III behavior in this illustration is determined as the expected outcome by the planners. Then judgments are made as to whether the cognitive or affective domain is to be the focal point. The decision may well be that all three levels are in the affective domain.

Likewise, a cognitive behavior may not begin in the cognitive domain but in the affective domain instead. An illustration was selected from the previous list of behaviors:

Level I   A2.3   The nursing student takes the initiative in seeking readings that increase the understanding of various sociocultural interpretations of the concepts of health and illness.

Level II   C3.0   The nursing student uses relevant sociocultural concepts of health and illness in assessing the health needs of a particular patient and family.

Level III   C4.2   The nursing student relates the patient's response to health or illness to sociocultural background.

Cognitive behaviors also may be developed only within the one domain, the cognitive. Because the taxonomy of the psychomotor domain is not fully developed at this point, it will not be used as part of this systematic approach. It would seem that the first four stages in the taxonomy formulated by Dave would evolve within a unit or course, depending upon the complexity of the skill. In this taxonomy, Level 5, naturalization, is comparable to Level 3, application for the cognitive domain, i.e., the ability to use the skill as a means rather than an end.

AFFECTIVE OBJECTIVES AND BEHAVIORS

The following are examples of affective behavioral objectives and their behaviors.

BEHAVIORAL OBJECTIVE

A. 3.1   The student provides opportunity for the hospitalized adult to express own beliefs, interests, and needs.

BEHAVIORS

A. 3.1   Accepts responsibility for listening to clients express ideas for plans of care

A. 3.1   Encourages client to express own concerns

A. 3.1   Considers client's preferences when supportive of his or her care

A. 3.0   Makes adjustments in nursing care to meet expressed needs of the client

A. 3.1   Supports the client's right to confidentiality

BEHAVIORAL OBJECTIVE

A.3.2   The student accepts responsibility for developing competence in carrying out a psychosocial assessment process

BEHAVIORS

C. 3.0   Identifies personal variables which influence the psychosocial assessment

C. 2.3   Determines own response to clients of varied cultural, religious, and sexual life styles

A. 3.2   Examines willingly own feelings about the data obtained in a
psychosocial assessment process

A. 3.2   Discusses with other nursing colleagues own feelings and
actions regarding the psychosocial assessment process

A. 3.2   Assumes responsibility for reviewing the literature and current research relating to psychosocial assessment

A. 3.2   Assumes responsibility for self-direction in obtaining assessment experiences as needed for reaching competency

THE DEVELOPMENTAL PROCESS IN BEHAVIORAL OBJECTIVES

The evolution of behavioral development within a program involves movement on a vertical plane through the system, as depicted in the model (Fig.
5-1), i.e., from program to lesson plan or individual learning experience
behavioral objectives, with feedback into the relevant subsystem.

The vertical movement assures a connection for all parts of the system,
thus certifying that goal development is continuous and consistent. This
means that the goals of each subsystem are compatible with each other,
contributing to the growth and development of each other as well as to the
total system.

Table 5-1 illustrates the vertical process in sequencing behavior, within a
baccalaureate nursing program, from the program level through individual
behaviors within a unit of the course. This illustration also shows the process
of value development, as discussed in a previous section of this chapter,
moving from cognitive to affective domain. In this example it is assumed that
the first nursing course is offered in the sophomore year.

As noted, the ultimate level of achievement expected for students in this
program is one in which valuing has achieved a systems organization. At the
junior-year level, value development is anticipated at the commitment stage
characterized by consistent behavior that would eventually be incorporated
into a value system. This means that all courses in the junior year should
contribute to this development. Consistency in behavior refers to respect for

TABLE 5-1

Behavioral Objectives Sequence—Program to Unit—Baccalaureate Program

System	Program (Senior Level)	A4.2	The nursing student interacts with others in a facilitative manner, reflecting value for the dignity and worth of each individual involved.
	Junior Level	A3.3	The nursing student respects the dignity of each individual involved in an interaction
Subsystem I	Sophomore Level	C3.0	The nursing student generalizes about the effect of values on interpersonal relationships
Subsystem II	Course: Human Relations	C2.3	The nursing student makes inferences relative to the effect of values on the interpersonal relationships
Subsystem III	Unit: Human Sexuality	C2.3	The nursing student determines the relationship between one's values and the concept of human sexuality
	Unit Behaviors	C2.2	Explains association between human relations concept and a concept of human sexuality
		C2.3	Differentiates between facts and myths or superstitions relating to sexual behavior
		C2.3	Differentiates values that are supportive in developing one's own sexual identity
		C2.3	Differentiates values that impede development of one's own sexual identity
		C2.3	Determines cultural factors that have influenced own concepts of human sexuality
		A2.2	Discusses willingly own values regarding human sexuality

all individuals, not only those with values and life styles similar to those of the student.

In the sophomore year the student focuses on the cognitive component of value development and, by the end of the year, should be able to generalize about prejudice relative to interpersonal relationships.

The illustration includes a course in Human Relations at the sophomore level. Since the behavioral objectives of the course are at a cognitive level of inference rather than the level of generalization as specified for the sophomore year, it may be assumed that the course is offered early in the sophomore year. One unit, Human Sexuality, anticipates cognitive development at the inference level.

Included below the unit behavioral objectives is a list representing individual behaviors the student must meet to demonstrate that the objective of the course has been achieved. These behaviors may be stated for individual learning experiences.

The important point in this illustration is that all parts of the system contribute to achieving the program behavioral objective. Units obtain their reference frame from courses, courses obtain their reference from a level, and levels are identified within the reference supplied by the program behavioral objective.

Table 5-2 shows a similar process of development for a two-year diploma or associate degree nursing program. The outcome is identified at the level of preference for a value. The first year of the program emphasizes the cognitive process, with the inference level of achievement anticipated. It will be noted that the course offered, Human Relations, is similar to that in the baccalaureate program, but an interpretation level of development is anticipated for students in this program.

The unit behavioral objective is also at the level of interpretation. A difference is noted between the unit behaviors listed for baccalaureate students and two-year nursing program students. Students in the latter program are geared to the interpretative and translation level of cognition, whereas baccalaureate students are to reach the inferential level of achievement.

Both illustrations, however, suggest a systematic approach to behavioral objective development, which combines the developmental model with the taxonomic concept. All levels are involved in the totality of and in the development of each part of the system. Continuity rather than disjunction characterizes the process, and the outcome can be evaluated easily when all parts of the system are directed toward the same goal.

The subsystems identified with staff development and continuing education programs depend on the framework in which they are defined. A process similar to the one proposed for programs in schools is in order because program objectives are developed throughout the system. The subsystems may bear different labels, but the process is the same.

TABLE 5-2

Behavioral Objectives Sequence—Program to Unit—Diploma or Associate Degree Program (Two Years)

System	Program (Second Level)	A3.2	The nursing student establishes interpersonal relationships based on respect for dignity and worth of each individual.
Subsystem I	First Level	C2.3	The nursing student predicts the effect of values on interpersonal relationships.
Subsystem II	Course: Human Relations	C2.2	The nursing student explains the relationship between values and interpersonal relationships.
Subsystem III	Unit: Human Sexuality	C2.2	The nursing student explains the relationship between one's values and human sexuality.
	Unit Behaviors	C2.2	Explains the association between interpersonal relations concepts and concepts of human sexuality
		C1.23	Names some commonly held myths and superstitions which relate to sexual behavior.
		C2.1	Gives illustrations of values which are supportive in developing one's sexual identity
		C2.1	Gives illustrations of values which impede the development of one's sexual identity
		C2.2	Explains cultural factors which have influenced own concept of human sexuality
		A2.2	Discusses willingly own values regarding human sexuality

USE OF SYSTEMS MODEL FOR LEVELING OBJECTIVES

The Systems Model (Fig. 5-1), based on Chin's developmental model, assumes that nursing education is a developmental process identifiable by specifically defined levels. A level is a point in the development scale which defines certain competencies to be achieved and demands that the teacher and learner be accountable for their attainment. If attainment has not been achieved, then a rationale must be provided from supporting data.

The use of the model implies that in a nursing education program, the learner's growth and development in relation to the competencies needed of a nurse practitioner become the critical variables in the program. The competencies defined as behavioral outcomes at each level are expressed in terms of directional progress goals, for all levels must ultimately contribute to the program objectives as defined by the faculty of a program.

It is essential that the program outcomes be realistic within the framework of the present educational system and the resources available to the faculty. Argyris and Schön (1974) warn us that "the school cannot claim the entire function of helping students to acquire professional competence—at least not without restructuring the concepts of school and office so that the traditional boundaries between them virtually disappear." As they address the incompatibilities between the time and experiences needed to develop professional competencies and the structure of school experiences such as course work, term papers, defined school terms, etc., they remind us that the intensity and duration of involvement in practice are too limited in educational programs to enable the student to acquire a full range of professional competence.[3]

Program objectives are general objectives which encompass behaviors in all domains: cognitive, affective, and psychomotor. The objectives are stated as outcomes (some people call these objectives *terminal*) and then specific behaviors are developed under each objective. These behaviors indicate what the student must accomplish in order to demonstrate attainment of the objective.

The delineation of program objectives for a nursing program is dependent upon the concept of nursing accepted by a faculty. Nursing, as perceived by this author, is a theoretically derived practice discipline based on a value system reflective of the inherent worth and dignity of an individual. This concept then suggests six possible areas which must be reflected in a set of program objectives of a nursing education program.

1. *Theory framework* of the curriculum, such as: adaptation, health field concept, needs, self-care, behavior systems, life process.

EXAMPLE: The student practices nursing within the adaptation framework as it relates to the client in all stages of development at any point on the health-illness continuum.

2. *Nursing methodology*—nursing process.

EXAMPLE: The student uses the nursing process in meeting the health care needs of clients.

3. *Concept of inherent worth and dignity of the individual*—may be stated as an objective or may be combined with another objective.

EXAMPLE: The student accepts responsibility to provide nursing care reflective of an individual client's inherent worth and dignity.

4. *Interrelationships*—often refers to intra- and inter-disciplinary interactions; may also refer to client interactions.

EXAMPLE: The student interacts in a facilitative, purposeful manner with clients, families, colleagues, and members of other health care disciplines.

5. *Student development*—toward self actualization.

EXAMPLE: The student develops a self-identity which supports continued development as a learner, nursing practitioner, and a contributing member of society.

6. *Profession*—relates to the practitioner and the profession as they interface with the health of society and patterns of health care organization.

EXAMPLE: The student identifies the dimensions of accountability of the nurse and the profession toward society as it seeks to meet health care needs of its constituents.

These six areas represent, for the most part, the dimensions of a basic program toward which development should be directed. It is important that not too many objectives be stated, for once the objectives become too specific, there is the real danger of exclusion of other equitable behaviors— that is, inclusion can often lead to exclusion. The behavioral level at which these objectives are designated and the complexity of variables with which these behaviors occur are determined by the type of educational program for which they have been developed.

Once the faculty has prepared the outcome objectives, they are leveled to indicate the progression in their development. The number of levels in a program is determined by the faculty. Many use years in a program as a framework for identifying levels. Levels must be of sufficient length of time for learning to occur, therefore, they should be limited in number for any particular educational program.

There are two ways in which leveling of objectives may be accomplished. The behavior itself may be changed to indicate a higher taxonomy level or the variables with which the behavior is to be carried out may be changed to indicate complexity. The ability to use the nursing process is more complex (i.e., higher level) than the ability to explain the nursing process. Likewise, the skills used in the nursing process with individuals are less complex than those used with groups.

With some leveling, only the behavior is changed; with others only the variables concerned with the behavior are altered; whereas in some instances both the behavior and variables are changed.

EXAMPLE: *Level I*
The student *explains* the nursing process as it relates to the care of a *patient*.

EXAMPLE: *Level II*
The student *uses* the nursing process to provide care to *the patient and his family*.

Leveling thus first involves the delineation of objectives as outcomes for the program. It is important to remember that since these objectives state the competencies expected at the conclusion of the program, they must be attainable and measurable. Therefore, they should not represent a projection of what the student will achieve as a graduate. The objectives cannot state an expectation that the student will be accountable for nursing practice as a professional nurse. The student, at the program's conclusion, is not a professional nurse. That behavior must be evaluated at a later time in a study of graduates.

It is also important to recognize that the objectives of the program are also the objectives of the last year of the program. If the objectives define expectations of competency at the conclusion of the program, that conclusion occurs at the end of the last year. There is no need for senior-level objectives in a program; they are already stated.

After these program objectives have been developed, the behaviors for each objective must be stated. These behaviors indicate the specific behaviors that the student will demonstrate to validate achievement of the objective. These behaviors also are subject to the leveling process.

SUMMARY

A systematic approach to the development of behavioral objectives is predicated on the assumption that a system (program behavioral objective) exists in which subsystems are included, namely, level, course, and unit behavioral objectives, as well as lesson plan and/or individual learning experience behavioral objectives. To assure the continuous development of expected outcomes, all subsystems must be connected with the system and must contribute to the expressed goals of the program.

Chin's developmental model serves as a framework, and the taxonomy provides the methodology for specifying various levels of behavior development in each subsystem as well as interrelationships within the system.

It is essential to identify behaviors where attainment constitutes achievement of objectives. As behavior development progresses during the program, stated behavioral objectives or behaviors may remain within one domain or change to another domain at any point in the system.

REFERENCES

1. Chin, R. The Utility of System Models and Developmental Models for Practitioners. In Bennis, W., Benne, K.& Chin, R. (eds): The Planning of Change, New York: Holt, Rinehart & Winston, 1961, p. 201.
2. *Idem:* p. 208.
3. Argyris, C. & Schön, D. Theory In Practice. Increasing Professional Effectiveness. San Francisco:Jossey-Bass, 1974, p. 186.

RECOMMENDED READINGS

Aiken, L. & Aiken, J. A Systematic Approach to the Evaluation of I.P.R. Am. J. Nurs., 73:863, 1973.

Bloom, B.S. (ed), Engelhart, M.D., Furst, E.J., Hill, W.H., & Krathwhol S.R. Taxonomy of Educational Objectives: Handbook I, Cognitive Domain. New York: David McKay, 1956.

Krathwohl, D.R., Bloom, B.S., & Masia, B.B. Taxonomy of Educational Objectives: Handbook II, Affective Domain. New York: David McKay, 1964.

6 Preparation of Behavioral Objectives for Continuing Education or Staff Development Programs

The preparation of behavioral objectives for continuing education and staff development programs occurs within a framework which is similar to, but also different from, that of the more formalized programs of study in a nursing school. For the most part, behavioral objectives for these programs are directed toward a narrow, specific area of nursing knowledge or practice offered within a short span of time. The technique of writing these behavioral objectives is the same as for all educational programs, but the limiting characteristic of continuing education and staff development programs challenges the program planner in relation to substance and outcome expectations.

In this chapter, the term *continuing education program* encompasses the concept of staff development programs. It is recognized that some nurse educators differentiate between these two types of programs, but a definition of a continuing education program which refers to an education program directed toward the learning needs of the practitioners would also include staff development programe.

BEHAVIORAL OBJECTIVES AS A CONTRACT

The statement of objectives for a continuing education program is in essence a contract with the consumer, for it tells that individual what is the expected outcome of that experience. The statement is one of the most important factors in influencing a consumer to participate in the program.

The increasing demand for continuing education programs to meet the needs of practitioners who must continuously update knowledge and practice competencies challenges program planners to develop programs that are relevant, worthwhile, and of high quality. Reilly (1976) states: "The institution of a requirement such as continuing education places demands upon constituents, employees, and the public. These demands are economic, social, temporal, intellectual, physical, and emotional. Because of the multifaceted nature of these demands, it is most important that program planners assure that their offerings merit the expenditures entailed."[1] Behavioral objectives stated clearly so as to define the focus of the program and a program plan consistent with the stated objectives must be communicated to the target population so that the membership will be informed as to what it is purchasing. Objectives are a significant component of continuing education programs. They are not a pedagogical exercise representing a skill in combining words and phrases into some fine sounding statement reflective of current fads in educational or nursing jargon. They are, instead, reflective statements of what is to be and must meet the test of "truth in advertising" demanded by consumers in all parts of our society. They communicate the intent and direction of the program and require the program planners to be held accountable for providing opportunities for the participants to obtain the objectives.

The statement of behavioral objectives does not guarantee that all participants will attain the objectives, for the achievement of any individual rests with that person's readiness and motivation to learn. The program planner is stating, however, that there will be opportunity provided to engage in the specified learning. The stated objectives enable the individual to have the knowledge of the learning to be achieved and the option to make the decision as to whether or not that learning is wanted or needed.

PURPOSE OF CONTINUING EDUCATION PROGRAMS

What is the goal of all continuing education programs in nursing? The position of the continuing educator is a recent innovation within professional schools and health care agencies. The early stages in the development of such a position in health care agencies provided solely for instruction in orientation of new personnel or on-the-job training for certain classifications of personnel. Universities and other institutions of higher learning focused their energies on moving nurses through the academic route with a degree as the sign of achievement. Although there were great pronouncements about the expanding knowledge base of nursing practice as new developments occurred in its related science fields, little emphasis was given to the need of the nurse in practice to update knowledge and competencies. When the need was recognized, many nursing continuing education programs followed the historical route and sought assistance from people outside the discipline.

Thus many programs were provided by doctors, pharmacists, educationists, psychologists, etc. Very few program planners called upon members of the nursing discipline to help the nurse broaden knowledge and competencies that led to greater depth in the nursing practice. It was also noted that while nursing has called upon these outside disciplines, nursing has not been asked to contribute to knowledge of the practitioners in those disciplines. The interdisciplinary teaching was unilateral.

These comments are not intended to suggest that all programs must be conducted by nurses: they are to suggest that our business is to assist with the practitioner's practice and that the contribution of various disciplines must be seen within that context, not as the source of the fulfillment of the continuing education needs of nursing practitioners.

The goal of continuing education programs must relate to the nature of the nursing discipline. Nursing is a theoretically derived practice discipline based on a value system reflective of man's inherent dignity and worth. What does this conceptualization of practice suggest to the program planners about the substance of the objectives they develop? It certainly identifies the nurse practitioner as a user of knowledge, especially as the profession is now developing its own generators of knowledge, the nurse researchers. However, most of the programs offered will be geared toward the in-depth preparation of the nurse as a user of knowledge by expanding the theory base and by helping with the development of problem solving and decision making skills as well as the varied assessment and intervention competencies.

SOURCES OF BEHAVIORAL OBJECTIVES

The critical question in the preparation of behavioral objectives for a program relates to the WHAT, the substance of the objectives. Where does one go to find the focus in order to be able to select the appropriate outcomes that are relevant to the target population for whom the program is designed?

There are four areas where competency is expected of any nurse practitioner today. These areas provide an excellent source for identifying the content of any continuing education offering.

1. A NURSING MODEL AS A FRAMEWORK FOR PRACTICE. This area is a relatively new dimension in nursing, yet it is a critical one if nursing is to define its own limits of practice. Theory development in nursing is making rapid strides toward an eventual nursing science. Currently nursing practice is moving within conceptual frameworks that describe nursing practice rather than predict it as a theory could. These frameworks are attempts to help nurses view their practice from a nursing perspective rather than from a medical model. What are continuing educators doing to help the nurse in practice understand the theory behind practice and the evolution of a nursing model?

Is this information to be maintained only for the new practitioners and the graduate prepared nurses located in universities? Do not current practitioners also need this new knowledge to impact their own actions?

2. NURSING PROCESS. This second area relates to the way one nurses. It addresses nursing's method of practice. It states that nursing is a problem-solving process demanding decision making and clinical judgment rather than being a task-oriented discipline as many perceive it to be. The process incorporates skills in data gathering, scientific interpretation, nursing diagnoses, intervention, and finally evaluation for determining both the outcome of care and the process by which the nurse arrived at the outcome. Every profession has its own method of operation. Nursing process is nursing's method. It represents all domains of action—cognitive, affective, psychomotor—within a moral and ethical framework. Continuing education programs need to focus on skill development in nursing process. Emphasis in programs on one aspect, such as physical assessment skills, without relating these skills to all other aspects of the process perpetuate the task approach to nursing.

3. INTERPERSONAL SKILLS. Nurses are in the people business. Competency in interacting with clients, families, colleagues, other disciplines, and the public is essential if nursing actions are to be effective. This area incorporates many focal points for evolving programs. The various theories, concepts, and processes as well as techniques and strategies are all legitimate areas of concern.

4. MEMBERSHIP IN A PROFESSION. This area is concerned with the responsibilities inherent in membership in a collective group—a profession. Concerns here relate not only to the nurse's own role but to the role of a profession within a worldwide community. Nursing practice is developed and functions within a professional framework. The focus of the behavioral objectives must also be relevant to that framework, especially in terms of the trends, movements, and future goals of that profession. The changing role of the nurse as newer health needs emerge, the interface of nursing with other health related disciplines, the economics of health care pertinent to payment for nursing services, issues about quality assurance programs for care, the legislative actions which relate to nursing practice and nursing education, and the credentialing of nursing's educational programs and services are all legitimate areas for the development of objectives.

Objectives must also reflect the issues, movements, and concerns of the society to which we belong. Although our professional sphere occupies a considerable portion of our life, neither that profession nor we as individuals live in a vacuum. We are constantly interfacing with many facets of our society and the clients we serve are of that society. Therefore, as behavioral objectives are prepared, they must reflect the real world. What are the implications of biases based on race, religion, sex, physical deformities, and age on the nurse's approach to the clients? What do inflation, violence, changing nature of family structure, consumer movements, and environmental issues have to do with the programs offered? Outcomes must be designed to help the nurse live and work within a changing society, where the absolutes of good and bad no longer apply with the certainty that many older practitioners remember. They must also be designed to assist the nurse in explaining the ethical, moral, and value issues which impinge on the nursing practice and influence the impact the practice will have on the health care of society.

Emphasis on the substance of the objectives has been stressed at this point to focus on the need for validity of objectives. A perfectly worded objective that is completely out of the realm of reality is of little use to one seeking continued education experiences. The variety of sources that the program planner goes to for the focus of the behavioral objectives will enable the individual to avoid getting into a rut with programs. Too often, program planners tend to have the subject matter of programs arise from a limited vision of their work world so that programs become repetitive and boring and do little to expand the horizons of the practitioners.

TARGET POPULATION

Continuing education programs are designed for a very specific population—adult learners who are primarily engaged in the practice of nursing. Employment means a continuing involvement in the practice which influences the nurse's decision as to need for further education. The origin of the need from the work setting may be a positive factor in that it provides a source of motivation for the nurse's involvement in the program. However, it may also be an impediment to the nurse's decision making, for the experience may have fostered "tunnel vision" so that the greater parameters of nursing practice may not be recognized. Program planners are then challenged to develop behavioral objectives that help these nurses recognize their own need to expand their perspective of nursing.

Knowledge of the characteristics of the population group is as essential for writing behavioral objectives for continuing education programs as it is for any other type of educational program. Employment variables must be included in the development of a group's profile, for there is a close relationship between area of practice and attendance at continuing education programs. The profile of the target population is particularly significant in planning learning behavior outcomes, for the level of achievement designated must be compatible with the background of the population.

Recognition of adult learning principles is especially significant as program objectives are developed. The adult learner's need to be involved in the learning process requires that objectives reflect action and participation.

Too many programs are really "show and tell." Experts come before a group to show their wares and tell what they know. The learner can choose how much or how little involvement is desired. With no provision for active involvement in the process, the adult learner becomes tuned out and frustrated in the effort to relate the new learning to individual experiences. The interest in problem solving, the search for fulfillment of individually designated goals, and the ability to be self-directing are essential attributes of the adult learner which must be addressed in any continuing education program planning and must be reflected in the objectives stated for the program.

WRITING OF BEHAVIORAL OBJECTIVES

The format for writing behavioral objectives as described in Chapter 3 remains the same for the behavioral objectives prepared for continuing education programs. The particular nature of these programs, however, demands special considerations in determining the outcome as identified in the selection of the behavioral verb.

Selection of Action Verb

One of the first considerations in writing the behavioral objectives is the selection of the appropriate verb to connote the intended behavioral outcome. The list of verbs identified for each level of the three taxonomies that appear in Chapter 4 is most useful in designating the outcome. These verbs make our objectives more precise in meaning and facilitate communication between the program planner and the target population. Because of the characteristics of the audience and the goal of continuing education programs to assist the nurse in using new knowledge, the verbs identified in the first level of the cognitive and affective domains would be inappropriate. Listing or defining behaviors is primarily recall and requires no comprehension of the phenomena described. The following objective is appropriate for users of knowledge at the graduate nurse level.

> *The learner relates ethical theories to the decisions nurses make within the context of their practice.*

The verb must also reflect a behavior that can be achieved within the limitations imposed by structure and time. Objectives that must be met outside the conference cannot be stated unless the program is a series extended over a period of time with practice planned for the intervening periods.

Example: The learner participates within the maternity nurse's professional role during the patient's delivery period.

It is most probable that this behavior could not be met in a workshop of a day or two. However, the conceptual behavior could be achieved.

The learner describes the professional role of the maternity nurse during the patient's delivery period.

The development of a skill to a certain level of competency within a one- or two-day workshop is also questionable. This time frame provides for practice in the skill, but skill development demands more than most such workshops can provide. A behavior, then, might reflect a process inherent in the workshop rather than a direct outcome.

The application skill as expressed by such verbs as *use* and *apply* are more appropriate for longer workshops, where time allows for practice. Some formats that call for a one- or two-day session followed by assignments to be carried out in the work setting and then a meeting at a later date may have objectives that are behaviorally expressed as application relative to nursing practice. If the workshop provides practice sessions with the use of such skills as communication, problem solving, and decision making, the behaviors may be expressed as application outcomes.

The following objective is most appropriate for a skill in a one- or two-day continuing education program.

The learner practices techniques appropriate to the assessment of the adult's nervous system.

There are times when the behavioral objectives for a short-term workshop will be expressed in terms of the process behaviors rather than the outcome behaviors. Terms appropriate for such objectives are:

challenge	interact
communicate with	participate
contribute	practice
examine	question
explore	share ideas, concerns, etc.

Number of Behavioral Objectives

The number of behavioral objectives appropriate for a program depends upon the intent of the program and its length. For most programs, the range of behavioral objectives is from four to six, a number which is most realistic for achievement, although even fewer objectives may be appropriate. At least one behavioral objective should be addressed to the relationship of the topic to nursing practice, for that legitimizes the program. The science theory is usually reflected in another behavior. Other objectives may relate to actual processes of the workshop activities such as *participates, explores, uses a problem-solving approach*, etc. Societal issues may also be indicated, and when psychomotor skills, interview skills, etc. are included, they need to be identified at the appropriate level of competency.

SUMMARY

The process of behavioral objective writing for continuing education programs represents many components, namely: the content to be addressed, the characteristics of the target population, the selection of action appropriate to the level of the learner and the time frame available, and the appropriateness of the objective to the nature of and setting of the continuing education offering. All of these components must be considered in preparing any set of objectives for a continuing education program.

Continuing education programs have special characteristics defined by their target population, which is composed of adult practitioners, and the limitations imposed by time and the scope of content restrictions. Their primary purpose is to facilitate the continued development of the practitioners and their practice. These characteristics demand that the program planner select appropriate behavioral objectives which are meaningful and achievable. Once the behavioral objectives are developed, they become a contract with the consumer and the continuing educator is accountable for developing a program congruent with the stated intent.

REFERENCES

1. Reilly, D.E. Preparation of Objectives for Continuing Education Programs. OCCH, Nurs., Vol. 14:12,30 December 1976.

RECOMMENDED READINGS

Argyris, C. & Schön D. Theory in Practice: Increasing Professional Effectiveness. San Francisco:Jossey-Bass, 1974.
Bigge, M.L. Learning Theories for Teachers. New York:Harper and Row, 1964.
Brown, B. (ed) Continuing Education—Who Cares? Nurs. Adminis. Quart., 2:1–82, Winter 1978.
Hutsch, D., Nesselroade, J. R. & Plemens, J.K. Learning Ability Relations in Adulthood, Human Dev., 19, 234–247, 1976.
Kidd, J.R. How Adults Learn. New York:Associated Press, 1976.
Knox, A.B. Adult Development and Learning. San Francisco:Jossey-Bass, 1977.
Lauffer, A. The Practice of Continuing Education in the Human Services. New York: McGraw-Hill Book Co., 1977.

Merriam, S. Middle Age: A Review of the Literature and Its Implications for Educational Intervention. *Adult Ed.*, Vol. 29, No. 1, 39–54, 1978.

Popiel, E.S. (ed) Nursing and the Process of Continuing Education (2nd ed). St. Louis:Mosby, 1977.

Rodgers, J. Adults Learning. Baltimore:Penguin Books, 1973.

Tobin, H.M., Wise P.Y. & Hull, M.K. Adult Learning in the Process of Staff Development Components for Change. St. Louis:Mosby, 1979.

Vermilye, Dyckman, W. (ed) Lifelong Learner—A New Clientele for Higher Education. San Francisco:Jossey-Bass, 1974.

7 Evaluation

Throughout the discussion of behavioral objectives, frequent reference was made to the relationship between objectives and evaluation. Behavioral objectives provide the WHAT and suggest clues for the HOW of evaluation, unless they are expressed as specific behavioral objectives. In this latter form, the specifics of the HOW are included in the behavioral objective.

In the vast amount of literature about educational evaluation, one concept that consistently appears is usually stated in the following manner: *evaluation is related to objectives* and is *delineated in terms of measurable student behavior*. Evaluation is a complex, multidimensional process, but the discussion in this book will be directed to that aspect of evaluation in an educational endeavor that is associated with behavioral objectives.

ATTITUDES TOWARD EVALUATION

Evaluation is a judgmental process and, as such, it reflects the beliefs, values, and attitudes of participants. A critical determinant of the direction of evaluation is how the evaluator defines the term *evaluation*. As previously stated, *value* is part of the word formation, and since value is a personal concept, evaluation must be subjective.

Within the educational system of our society, evaluation has ordinarily been associated with grading performance and classifying students. More will be said later about the differences between these two processes. Since many associate evaluation with grading and classifying individuals and since our society uses these grades and/or classifications for many purposes, nurse teachers are asked to assume an awesome responsibility. Their judgment of a learner influences the student's job opportunities, choice of a career, acceptance and continuation in a program of studies, and even the student's social and personal identity within the matrix of society itself. As evaluators, faculty and other teachers in nursing are in a position to influence the destiny of learners with whom they are involved.

One significant question must be answered by each nurse teacher, because the response determines the approach taken toward evaluation. Is evaluation a process for growth, or is it a means for control? The answer will come from the teacher's beliefs about man, the nature of the learner, and the nature of the teaching-learning process. The answer also will determine whether the teacher will ask the right questions and see the right behavior with respect to the learning experience.

Present use of evaluation in our society supports a negative connotation. As a result, we find that the behaviors accompanying evaluation reflect:

anxiety instead of anticipation
punishment instead of reward
defeatism instead of encouragement
compliance instead of self-determination
safety instead of risk-taking

Many nurse teachers support the premise that a primary goal in living is the individual's ability to know the self and to develop progressively to fulfill his/her potential. Evaluation is a major process in helping the individual to achieve self-actualization, yet as customarily used, evaluation has not consistently helped others to realize this goal. Instead, self-knowledge may be considered so frightening that a defensive approach to evaluation becomes a common pattern of behavior.

No doubt evaluation carries a strong power component and use of this power is circumscribed by the evaluator's perception of the process. Some individuals have a consistent need to control others, thus evaluation can be a potent weapon. Unfortunately, all helping professions appear to attract these "controllers of man," for these professions concern themselves with individuals or groups who are more or less dependent. Controllers base their evaluation on rules, regulations, and procedures, tending to manipulate the learner in order to fit behavior into the accepted code. Learners are then forced to direct their energies toward surviving in the system, rather than toward experiences that would contribute to growth and development.

The power component, however, also is used by evaluators who are facilitators and who perceive evaluation as related to the learner's growth. These individuals accept the concept of mastery of learning, and, by using evaluation as a diagnostic process, develop teaching strategies that stimulate the learner to search for self-knowledge and to develop his/her potential. Rules, regulations, and procedures are not ends in themselves but means to ends that best serve the learner and other persons in a particular setting.

The power potential in evaluation also affects evaluators who perceive the process in terms of themselves rather than as a growth process for the student whereby progress is made toward achieving behavioral objectives. The student's success or failure is equated with the teacher's success or failure. If students succeed, it goes unnoticed, but if a student fails, the teacher responds as though the failure were a personal one. Guilt, self recrimination, and depression are often the result.

In this situation, the teacher assumes his/her role is omnipotent. A belief in mastery of learning approach does not mean complete success for all students, because many variables associated with learning, including motivation and persistence, are ostensibly controlled by the learner. Failure requires an honest appraisal of all factors impinging on the teaching-learning process in order to establish a diagnosis and develop a suggested prescription for treatment. The diagnosis may indeed suggest faculty failure, or student failure, or even failure resulting from extraneous sources beyond the control of student or teacher.

CONCEPT OF THE PROCESS

Evaluation was defined previously as a process concerned with determining the quality of a substance, action, or event. In the context of education, evaluation refers to a process or combination of processes whereby nurse teachers judge student accomplishments relative to specific behavioral objectives.

Bloom, Hastings, and Madaus[1] (1971) express the following views about evaluation that connote the major purposes:

1. Evaluation as a method of acquiring and processing the evidence needed to improve student learning and teaching.
2. Evaluation as including a great variety of evidence beyond the usual final paper and pencil examination.
3. Evaluation as an aid in clarifying the significant goals and objectives of education and as a process of determining the extent to which students are developing in these desired ways.
4. Evaluation as a system of quality control in which it may be determined at each step in the learning process whether the process is effective or not, and if not, what changes must be made to insure its effectiveness before it is too late.

5. Evaluation as a tool in educational practice for ascertaining whether or not alternative procedures are equally effective in achieving a set of educational ends.

These views depict a vibrant, dynamic, continuous, open-ended process closely interwoven with the teaching-learning process. They are in sharp contrast to the all-too-frequently expressed view of evaluation as synonymous with grading or ranking students. The rationale for evaluation relates to assessment for growth: growth of the learner, growth of the teacher, growth of the teaching-learning process, and ultimately growth of the program and the institution offering the program.

Evaluation is not an end in itself, it is a means to an end. The process can enhance the students' personal development and learning or destroy the capacity to learn and distort personality development. Teachers should use evaluation wisely, consistent with developmental concepts of teaching-learning.

Two terms regarding evaluation are in current use today—summative evaluation and formative evaluation. Summative evaluation occurs at the end of a program, course, or unit, and refers to the extent to which the learner has realized all of specified behavioral objectives. Formative evaluation occurs throughout the program, course, and unit, and refers to the learner's progress toward realizing behavioral objectives. It states what is and what can be.

Summative evaluation is the more common practice in many programs; it is used to determine grades, certify students, and sometimes to judge the teacher's effectiveness. Tests or papers at midterm or final periods are the usual procedures. In this type of evaluation, there is a concept of finality, stating what is rather than what is combined with what can be.

The concept of formative evaluation is generally accepted in principle by many teachers, but a gap exists between expressed belief and action. This type of evaluation operates throughout the learning process and is concerned with the learner's progress during the learning period, not at the end of it. Formative evaluation relies on feedback to guide the learner and the teacher to aspects of learning that need critical attention as the learner moves toward mastery of the behavior. Varieties of evaluation procedures may be used. These include written tests, problem situations, observation of practice behaviors, conferences, and videotaping. The important point is that these procedures are not designed for grading a student but to assess progress, to diagnose learning needs so that remedial measures can be instituted promptly, and to pace the student's learning to individual needs and abilities. At the present time, formative evaluation is used sporadically in nursing programs and is usually directed to the poor student. A commitment to evaluation as an integral part of the teaching-learning process requires that a systematic approach to formative evaluation be developed and that summative evaluation be used periodically.

PSYCHOSOCIAL CLIMATE OF EVALUATION

Evaluation is presented as a positive process whose primary purpose is to assess growth. But, it was previously noted that many individuals involved in education do not view evaluation in this light. Practice, then, often has not been congruent with the belief that evaluation is a process directed toward development. How might participants in the teaching-learning process enjoy a positive experience in evaluation?

The critical variable in evaluation is the psychosocial climate prevailing during the process. The climate includes beliefs, values, feeling tones, and attitudes regarding evaluation of participants and the nature of the relationships existing among them. Rogers[2] (1969) refers to the attitudinal qualities of interpersonal relationships between facilitator and learner when he states:

> *First of all is a transparent realness in the facilitator, a willingness to be a person, to be and live the feelings and thoughts of the moment. When this realness includes a prizing, a caring, a trust, and respect for the learner, the climate for learning is enhanced. When it includes a sensitive and accurate empathic listening, then, indeed, a freeing climate stimulative of self initiated learning and growth exists. The student is TRUSTED to develop.*

Because evaluation is an integral part of the teaching-learning process, it significantly facilitates learning. The learning climate described by Rogers is relevant to the evaluation climate. The above quotation can be paraphrased to make it specific to this presentation.

> *First of all is a transparent realness in the* teacher evaluator, *a willingness to be a human being, to be and live the feelings and thoughts of the moment. When this realness includes a prizing, a caring, a trust, and respect for the learner, the climate for* evaluation *is enhanced. When it includes a sensitive and accurate empathic listening, then indeed a freeing climate stimulative of self-initiated* evaluation *and growth exists. The student is TRUSTED to develop.*

Maintaining the climate proposed by Rogers depends on the teacher's actions in the situation, for it is through actions that the student is able to assess the teacher's intent. One action that provides this facilitative environment for the evaluation experience is the use of behavioral objectives.

Behavioral objectives communicate to the learner the behaviors expected to be to developed and on which evaluation is to be based. If, in evaluating the student, the teacher adheres to the intent of the behavior, the student is free to learn and does not need to expend energy on outsmarting the instructor in preparation for evaluation. Behavioral objectives discipline the teacher to evaluate only the behavior indicated in the contract with the student. Thus, the teacher cannot focus on extraneous behaviors in an assessment, and teacher hang ups or biases are excluded. How often have evaluations of the nurse's behavior in a clinical practice setting paid minimal heed to competency in clinical practice but included numerous comments relative to length of hair, length of uniform, posture, etc. Evaluations of this latter type do much to undermine the climate of trust, and force the learner into playing games in an effort to survive. The survival need, and not the learning need, becomes the motivating force.

The climate described by Rogers predicates an environment in which learning includes opportunity for intelligent risk-taking. A developmental learning experience must provide students with opportunities to explore ideas and methods. A climate that values safety discourages the inquiring student, for the risks at evaluation time are too great. Rewards may be based on the results of the endeavor rather than on the process involved in the endeavor. Thus, the creative learner who dares to move from the tried path often is evaluated by a standard that frequently incorporates the utilitarian concept, "Is it workable?"

In too many instances, nurse teachers are uncomfortable with intelligent risk-taking, and safety is the predominating criterion used in providing student learning experience. Safety as referred to in this instance is unrelated to the reality of the situation and is usually a reflection of the teacher's insecurity. Intelligent risk-taking means the decision to take a novel action after the consequences of such an action have been considered. In most learning endeavors there is room for error, and, indeed, learning from mistakes is a creditable concept. Nursing programs, however, seek perfection in practice and allow little margin for error in the learning situation. Fear of error again restrains the learner from developing potential, for a record of errors becomes the content of many evaluations.

Prather[3] (1970) provides some insight into the role of mistakes in an individual's development.

Perfection is slow death. If everything were to turn out just like I would want it to, just like I would plan for it to, then I would never experience anything new; my life would be an endless repetition of stale successes. When I make a mistake I experience something unexpected.

I sometimes react to making a mistake as
if I have betrayed myself. My fear of making
a mistake seems to be based on the hidden
assumption that I am potentially perfect and
that if I can just be very careful, I will
not fall from heaven. But a "mistake" is a
declaration of the way I AM, a jolt to the
way I intend, a reminder I am not dealing with
facts. When I have listened *to my mistakes,*
I have grown.

Can students listen to their own mistakes? Are nurse teachers secure enough to permit students to listen to their mistakes? Formative evaluation should support the student's listening and help in finding new directions. A formative evaluation based on a concept of perfection is not one that supports the student in the search for self-knowledge and in developing potential. A climate in which mistakes are permitted to occur and provision is made for intelligent risk-taking as part of the learning process must be characterized by respect, trust, realness, and caring about the participants. It is under these conditions that evaluation can be accepted as a component of the teaching-learning process.

DIFFERENCES BETWEEN THE GRADING AND THE EVALUATION PROCESSES

Reference has been made to the fact that evaluation often is equated with grading. Frequently, when various types of evaluation procedures are discussed, the question is raised: How does one arrive at a grade from each procedure? Yet the concept of formative evaluation is not based on the premise of grading, but rather concerns itself with assessment for learner's guidance. Thus, all evaluation cannot be translated into grades.

Evaluation and grading are two separate processes. Whereas evaluation has been described as the process by which teachers make judgments about student achievement of designated behavioral objectives, grading is the process by which teachers assign symbols that represent the student's level of academic achievement. Grading has a quantitative dimension; evaluation has a qualitative dimension. The grading process then follows the evaluation process.

Grading is generally associated with summative evaluation, and translation of results of the evaluation is the most significant phase in the grading process. Unless the grade conveys sufficient information when it is interpreted, it has little value. The data base for any grade consists of whatever kinds of evidence a particular faculty member determines are indicators of student achievement as defined by that teacher. These components are then weighted and combined into a single scale by some formula developed by the faculty member. A symbol is then designated according to the student's placement on the scale. In reference to grades, Warren[4] (1971) says:

> Grades may therefore be accurate in reflecting performance on some undefined dimension of academic achievement. But their fidelity is poor in that they transmit only a small part of the information in the evaluations that led to the grade, while leaving the information they do transmit difficult to interpret.

Unfortunately, in too many instances the grading and the evaluation processes are too often considered synonymous. Erickson and Bluestone[5] (1971) state:

> The universal equation of grades and excellence does not escape the student; he works (not necessarily learns) for them as he registers his futile protest against being marked for life by a set of mysterious code letters. Whether by design or circumstance, the grade itself becomes a yardstick by which one student is measured against others; by its very simplicity, a transcript of grades encourages society to form simplistic judgments on a student's potential.

The issues relative to grading and its place in higher education are beyond the limits of this book. The discussion presented here is meant to clarify the difference between the evaluation and the grading processes, the former as a judgment of quality and the latter as a quantitative measurement. It is important for faculty to realize that the grade is ordinarily not a reliable and valid basis for evaluating a student's performance unless accompanied by a teacher's descriptive evaluation of the student's achievement.

NEED FOR A VARIETY OF EVALUATION STRATEGIES

It has been pointed out that evaluation is an integral part of the teaching-learning process and that it contributes to the learner's development. Because it is interwoven in the student's total educational experiences, a variety of approaches must be used. No one evaluation strategy is sufficient for all learners in all situations.

The following are five significant reasons for providing diversity in evaluation strategies.

1. COMPLEXITY OF HUMAN BEHAVIOR. Human behavior is a phenomenon representing the motivations, values, needs, experiences, and percep-

tions of an individual at any point in time. It is variable, changeable, open-ended, and responsive to stimuli from both the internal and external environment. Any process for appraising behavior must reflect recognition of its multidimensional character and include suitable methods that consider its complexity.

2. INDIVIDUAL DIFFERENCES IN RESPONSE TO LEARNING. Each individual's response to learning reflects one's abilities, interests, experiences, values, needs, beliefs, motivations, and perceptions. The learner has developed an individual style of learning and has become selective in the types of stimuli responded to in a learning situation. In any learning experience, no two individuals are alike in all dimensions. Evaluation processes, then, must provide for individual responses to any learning situation.

3. SUITABILITY OF SPECIFIC EVALUATION APPROACHES TO SPECIFIC TYPES OF LEARNING BEHAVIORS. Learning behaviors have been classified within three domains: cognitive, affective, and psychomotor. Each of these domains calls upon different abilities in the learner and requires different strategies for determining its behavioral attainment. As an example, an observation evaluation strategy is more appropriate for identifying a psychomotor competency than is a response on written paper.

4. MOTIVATIONAL FACTOR OF EVALUATION. Evaluation, especially formative evaluation, is designed to help the learner improve performance while still in the process of learning the behavior designated by the behavioral objective. It relies upon feedback to help both the teacher and the learner diagnose learning needs and intervene with appropriate teaching strategies. Evaluation that uses feedback and involves the learner in the appraisal is a significant factor in helping the learner to become self-motivating. Again, the use of various methods (especially in terms of the focus of the evaluation and the individuality of the student) can be helpful in the student's perception of the evaluation process as a means for self growth.

5. CREATIVE DIMENSION TO THE EVALUATION PROCESS. Like other teaching and learning strategies, evaluation strategies are most open to the teacher's and learner's creativity. An open-ended system of teaching promotes the acceptance of novelty in evaluation approaches to behavioral objectives, which often add vitality to the process. In too many instances, evaluation procedures are embedded in the "cement" of the educational program and become boring to students and teachers. In creating new evaluation methods or protocols, risk-taking plays an integral part. Sharing in a new venture can be a stimulating

experience to both students and teachers, especially if all are involved in assessing the evaluation strategy itself. Evaluation practices need not be in a rut; they can be creative, and therefore limited only by the extent of the imagination of participants and by their perseverance in pursuing the development, implementation, and assessment of practices.

The challenge then rests with the teacher who must develop and use evaluation strategies that are meaningful, relevant, and stimulating to the learner.

SUMMARY

Evaluation is the process or combination of processes whereby a teacher judges a student's accomplishment relative to specified behavioral objectives. The psychosocial climate in which this process occurs influences the effectiveness of the process. An environment characterized by respect, trust, empathy, caring, and risk-taking facilitates the evaluation process as an integral part of the teaching-learning process geared toward student growth and development. An environment created by individuals who need to control others fosters the use of evaluation as a force of control and directs student energy into game playing for survival rather than into learning pursuits.

Two types of evaluation are in current use. Formative evaluation occurs throughout the program, course, or unit, and through feedback enables teacher and student to diagnose learning needs, to provide appropriate remedial strategies, and to pace the student's learning according to his needs and abilities. Summative evaluation occurs at the end of the program, course, or unit and is concerned with the extent to which the learner has mastered all designated behavioral objectives. It is usually associated with grading but is not synonymous with it. Summative evaluation relates to the judgment a teacher makes about student achievement, whereas grading is the process by which the teacher assigns symbols that represent specific levels of student achievement.

Since evaluation is inherent in an effective teaching-learning process, varieties of strategies are indicated. Reasons for this variety are:

1. Complexity of human behavior.
2. Individual differences in learning.
3. Suitability of specific evaluation approaches to specific types of learning.
4. Motivational factor in evaluation.
5. The creative dimension to the evaluation process.

REFERENCES

1. Bloom, B.S., Hastings, J.T. & Madaus, G.F. Handbook on Formative and Summative Evaluation of Student Learning. New York:McGraw-Hill, 1971, p. 8.
2. Rogers, C. Freedom to Learn. Columbus, Ohio:Charles E. Merrill, 1969, p. 126.
3. Prather, H. Notes to Myself. Moab, Utah:Real People Press, 1970.
4. Warren, J. College Grading Practices: An Overview. Washington, D.C.:ERIC Clearinghouse on Higher Education, 1971, p. 2.
5. Erickson, S.C. & Bluestone, B.Z. Grading and Evaluation; Memo to the Faculty. Ann Arbor, Michigan:Center for Research on Learning and Teaching, 1971, p. 2.

RECOMMENDED READINGS

Anderson, S., Scarvia, B. & Ball, S. The Profession and Practice of Program Evaluation. San Francisco:Jossey-Bass, 1978.

Cooley, W.H. & Lohnes, P.R. Evaluation Research in Education: Theory, Principles and Practice. New York: Irvington, 1976.

Fivars, G. & Gosnell, D. Nursing Evaluation: The Problem and the Process. New York:Macmillan, 1966.

Green, J.L. & Stone, J.G. Curriculum Evaluation Theory and Practice. New York: Springer, 1977.

Mager, R.F. Goal Analysis. Belmont, California:Lear Siegler/Fearon, 1972.

Meleis, A.L. & Benner, P. Process or Produce Evaluation? Nurs. Outl., 23:303, 1975.

National League for Nursing: Evaluation—An Objective Approach: Report of the 1971 Workshops of the Council of Diploma Programs. New York:National League for Nursing, 1972.

National League for Nursing: Some Objective Approaches to Evaluation. New York: National League of Nursing, 1972.

Pace, C.R. (ed) New Directions for Higher Education: Evaluating Learning and Teaching. San Francisco:Jossey-Bass, 1973.

Pilehe, P. Delivery Puts Behavioral Objectives into Perspective. J. Nurs. Educ. Vol. 15. 5:7, September 1976.

Report of Ad Hoc Committee to Study Grading (unpublished). Detroit: Wayne State University, College of Nursing, 1973.

Sanford, N. (ed) American College. New York:Wiley, 1962.

Scriven, M. Evaluation Perspectives and Procedures. In Popham, W.J. (ed): Evaluation in Education: Current Applications. Berkeley:McCutchan, 1974.

Scriven, M.S. The Methodology of Evaluation. In Perspectives of Curriculum Evaluation. AERA Monograph Series on Curriculum Evaluation. No. 1, Chicago:Rand McNally & Co., 1967.

Suchman, E.A. Evaluative Research. New York:Russell Sage Foundation, 1967.

8 Methods of Evaluating Attainment of Behavioral Objectives

Behavioral objectives are the substance of evaluation in educational programs. They specify the behavior to be evaluated and the content to which the behavior is related. The point is that there must be a direct connection between the behavioral objective and the evaluation procedure.

The evaluation procedure must be addressed to the WHAT of the behavioral objective. One of the first steps in assuring this relationship is to select an evaluation method that provides data relative to the student's achievement of the designated behavior. The evaluation method must be appropriate to a particular situation.

A second step, however, is to determine whether the evaluation procedure really tests the behavior under examination. The method of evaluation may indeed be appropriate for a particular behavior, but the task implied in the method may be unrelated to the behavior. A written essay question on a test may be selected as the methodology for evaluating the nursing student's competency in explaining a concept of the nursing process. But if the task implied in the written question calls upon the student to list the steps in the process, the behavior of *explaining* is not being evaluated.

This chapter is concerned with the relationship between the WHAT and HOW of evaluation. Various methods of evaluation suitable to nursing programs are discussed and illustrated in relation to specific behavioral objectives. In the following examples, the learner in the objectives is the nursing student and only the behavior will be stated. The nursing student refers to any learner in nursing, i.e., a student in a school of nursing, or a practitioner in a staff development program or a program of continuing education. The coding before each behavior refers to the taxonomies discussed in Chapter 4.

PAPER AND PENCIL TEST ITEMS

Alternate Response

Test items in this classification ask the student to match one meaning of a fact, idea, concept, convention, or definition with the one presented. The student is asked to accept or reject the statement given. Forms of alternative response generally used are: true-false, accept-not accept, agree-disagree.

This form of test item is used most often in relation to the recall level of cognition. It is also effective in ascertaining beliefs and attitudes, the awareness or responding level of the affective domain. When students are directed to explain a rationale or defend a choice, the comprehensive level of cognition is being evaluated.

GENERAL PRINCIPLES OF CONSTRUCTION

The following are principles of construction:

1. The directions for answering the questions must be exact.
2. The truth or falsity should be expressed between subject and verb, never by a phrase tacked on at the end or by inserting an incidental phrase in the question.
3. The statement itself should be confined to one idea.
4. Specific determiners such as always, never, usually, generally, should be avoided.
5. There should be approximately the same number of false and true items.
6. A double space between items provides for easier reading.
7. Modifications can help to eliminate guessing. Suggestions include:
   a. explanation of false statement
   b. statement of reason for choice
   c. correction and/or revision of incorrect statement

ILLUSTRATIONS

BEHAVIORAL OBJECTIVES   TEST ITEM

Directions: For each of the following statements, circle "T" if the statement is true and "F" if the statement is false.

BEHAVIORAL OBJECTIVES	TEST ITEM
C1.25 Identifies primary sources of data collection for assessment of patient needs.	T.F. Consultation and patient interview are two primary sources of data collection relative to patient needs.
C1.32 Identifies the relationship between a pathological state and the signs and symptoms exhibited.	T.F. A decrease in breath sounds occurs in a condition such as atelectasis.
C1.11 Defines terminology referent to diseases of the heart.	T.F. Endocarditis is an inflammation of the heart muscle.

(If evaluation is to be addressed to the cognitive level of comprehension, the following statement is added to the instructions: In the space below each statement cite the rationale for your choice.)

C2.2 Differentiates between fact and stereotype about elderly people.	T.F. Old people are senile, ill, and nonproductive.
C2.2 Explains the relationship between oxygen concentration and physiological response.	T.F. Oxygen therapy in severe emphysema may result in apnea.

(If evaluation is to be addressed to the affective domain, the terms agree-disagree are used. The instructions then ask to circle the "A" or "D" instead of the "T" or "F".)

A1.1 Is aware that each individual has the right to quality nursing care.	A.D. The quality of nursing care needed for the substance abuser is different from that required by a college professor who is not a substance abuser.
A1.2 Acknowledges rights of patients.	A.D. Patients have the right to make decisions related to their plan of care.

Alternate response items are useful in testing a large area of content within a short period. They are easy to score unless an explanation is requested. They are useful in testing attitudes, misconceptions, and beliefs. In questions such as the ones listed above for the affective domain, responses should not be translated into grades. These kinds of questions are particularly good as part of the system of formative evaluation. Alternate response questions are subject to responses in which there is a large element of guessing unless the question requires justification for the response selected.

Multiple Recognition Questions

This format for questions provides students with several alternatives from which to choose the correct response. It is useful for the first three levels of cognition (knowledge, comprehension, and application) as well as for the first three levels in the affective domain (awareness, responding, and valuing). This format can be used in matching terms, definitions, generalizations, words, and systems as well as in conjunction with maps, diagrams, and charts.

There are two forms for this type of question.

1. Multiple choice: one answer is selected from a number of plausible ones. It may be the one *correct* answer, the best of several *correct* answers, or the one *incorrect* answer.
2. Multiple response: several correct responses are possible, and the selection is based on the best combination of responses.

GENERAL PRINCIPLES OF CONSTRUCTION

The following are principles of construction:

1. Structure: statement (stem) and a list of responses (alternatives or distractors)
2. Forms of statement
   a. Incomplete sentence relying on the alternative to complete it
   b. Complete statement
   c. Question
3. Forms of distractors
   a. Single word
   b. Phrase
   c. Complete sentence
4. Principles regarding the statement
   a. The statement must include the nature of the response:
      Which of the following *responses, functions, etc.* (do not just say which of the following)
   b. If only one response is desired—state which *one* of the following (functions).
   c. If the statement is to be completed by the response, do not place a period at the end of the statement. The period is placed after each response.

    d. Do not end an incomplete statement with *a* or *an* as this may give a clue to the correct response (*an* indicates a distractor beginning with a vowel).

    e. If statement asks for a response that does not apply—underline the word *NOT or EXCEPT* in the stem.

5. Principles regarding the response

    a. In any one question the response format must be consistent (i.e., all phrases, all one word, all complete sentences).

    b. If the response completes a statement, the first word of the response is in lower case and a period is at the conclusion of the response.

    c. If the response completes a statement, all responses must complete the statement grammatically.

    d. At least four responses should be included in any question.

    e. All responses should be logical and relevant to the statement.

    f. Responses that are obviously wrong or inappropriate weaken the questions.

    g. No response should give a clue to the answer.

    h. All responses should be placed at the conclusion of the statement.

SPECIAL CONSIDERATIONS RE MULTIPLE RESPONSE

1. Responses are generally identified as a letter.
2. The best combination of responses are identified by number. Instructions ask testee to circle the appropriate *number* preceding the best combination of responses.
3. There should be four or five combinations of responses.
4. In the combination, it is important that there be reasonable equity in selecting responses. Predominance in use of one letter or limited use of a letter provides clues to correct response.
5. It is advisable to indent the alternatives and to line up the combination of responses with the statement.

BEHAVIORAL OBJECTIVES

Multiple Choice

C2.2 Distinguishes abnormal from normal body change in the aging process.

TEST ITEM

Instruction: Circle the letter preceding the process that correctly completes the following statement.

The body change which is *not* a usual characteristic of aging is:

A. decrease in metabolism

BEHAVIORAL OBJECTIVES   **TEST ITEM**

B. loss in weight
C. loss of skin turgor
D. decrease in sensory function
E. frequency in urination

C1.22   Names the steps of the nursing process.

Instruction: Circle the letter preceding the correct sequence of steps in the nursing process.

The sequence of steps in the nursing process includes:
A. evaluation, planning, assessment, intervention
B. intervention, planning, evaluation, assessment
C. assessment, planning, intervention, evaluation
D. assessment, intervention, planning, evaluation

A3.1   Responds supportively to parents' expressed concern about their child's care.

Instruction: Circle the letter preceding the best response to the parents' expressed concern.

Mary, a two-year-old, is receiving I.V. therapy and is restrained. Her father says to you, "I know she needs fluids, but I hate to see her tied up like this." Your best response is:
A. "She is restrained for her own good so she won't pull out the needle."
B. "We restrain all the children receiving I.V.s."
C. "It is hard to see Mary restrained like this. The restraint is used so she will not dislodge the I.V. accidentally."
D. "We don't want her to pull out the I.V."

BEHAVIORAL OBJECTIVES	TEST ITEM

C1.21 Identifies physiological actions of exercise of joints.

Instruction: Circle the number preceding the best selection of responses.

Which of the following physiological actions occur with exercise of the knee?
A. Blood circulation is increased
B. Muscle tone is improved
C. Sensation in joints is lessened
D. Contractures are prevented
E. Mobility of joints is improved

1. All but C
2. B, D, E
3. All of the above
4. A, C
5. A, C, E

Multiple Response

C2.2 Detects clues in communication that connote a cultural interpretation of the time and/or space dimension.

Instruction: Circle the number preceding the best combination of responses.

Which of the following statements contain clues indicative of cultural interpretation of time and/or space?
A. "Yes, I will be available for an hour."
B. "Since the party starts at 6:30, I will invite him for 6:00."
C. "Don't touch me."
D. "Anyone who has to get that close to speak to someone has something wrong."

1. A, B, C
2. All of the above
3. All but A
4. A, B, D
5. A, C, D

BEHAVIORAL OBJECTIVES	TEST ITEM

A3.1   Supports individual in expressing grief.

Instruction: Circle the number preceding the best combination of responses.

Since Ms. D was notified that there is now lung involvement from metastases of her breast cancer, she has become withdrawn and speaks only when spoken to. Which of the following goals would you set for your nursing intervention?

A. Respect Ms. D's right to be silent
B. Protect patient from becoming emotionally upset
C. Encourage patient to talk about her feelings regarding her illness
D. Keep patient from morbidly dwelling on her illness
E. Keep staff informed as to the patient's method of handling her illness

1. A, C, E
2. All but D
3. C, D, E
4. All of the above
5. A, B, D

Multiple recognition questions, like alternate choice questions, are useful in testing large areas of content. This form is used widely in our educational system, but its use for making inferences about students is challenged by such educators as Barr (1963) and Hoffman (1962). Hoffman[1], in his thesis regarding the undesirability of multiple recognition questions, argues:

1. *The bright, creative students are particularly distracted by the ambiguity and oversimplification that, of necessity, result when ideas and concepts are confined to the restricted format of these types of questions. The better student, who often can see more in the question than is stated, is penalized.*
2. *The requirement of choosing the answer from among decoys does not reward intellectual honesty and thoroughness, but rather it places emphasis on skill in handling the type of question. Becoming test-wise*

is the result, instead, of demonstrating achievement of the objective for which the item is designed.

The student who sees more options than those provided in the question is required to play the game, unless provided with the opportunity to comment on the question to justify the choice of response.

Completion Questions

These questions require students to complete a statement by inserting the missing words or phrases. The format may be sentences or paragraphs. This format is primarily for the recall level of cognition with reference to definitions, specific terms, and technical terms.

GENERAL PRINCIPLES OF CONSTRUCTION

1. Blanks used at the end of a sentence simplify scoring.
2. Too many blanks in a statement should be avoided as the question could become puzzling.
3. All blanks should be standard length.
4. Key words are the ones to be omitted.
5. The use of *a* or *an* immediately preceding a blank should be avoided.
5. Only one answer should be possible for each blank.

BEHAVIORAL OBJECTIVES	TEST ITEM
	Instruction: Complete the blanks.
C1.12 Names community resources designed to meet the needs of mentally retarded children and their families.	Two community resources available to the parents of mentally retarded children are _____ and _____.
C1.11 Identifies a concept of integrity.	According to Erikson, the ability to look back on one's life with satisfaction is indicative of the achievement of _____.
C1.24 Identifies characteristics of sounds elicited when using auscultation technique.	The clear, long, low-pitched sound elicited over the normal lung is called _____.

Completion questions are useful in testing facts, but care must be taken that the blanks do not lead to ambiguity or to confusion so that the student is prevented from getting the sense of the statement. Some educators feel that this type of question fosters rote memorization in the learning process.

Matching Questions

Like other forms of questions discussed so far, this is an approach that provides for proficiency in terms of covering the content area of study. In this approach, the student is asked to relate facts, ideas, principles, or terms in one column to a statement or term in another column. Its primary use is in the recall process of cognition.

GENERAL PRINCIPLES OF CONSTRUCTION

1. Terms used should be stated clearly.
2. More choices should be listed in the right-hand column than things to be identified in the left-hand column. This eliminates the possibility of making choices by a process of elimination.
3. The terminology in the left-hand column should not give clues to the expected response in the right-hand column.
4. If each term in the right-hand column can be used more than once, this information should be included in the instructions.
5. The response list should be homogeneous in format.

Illustration

BEHAVIORAL OBJECTIVE

C1.2 Defines the terms of techniques used in a physical examination.

— 1. Percussion

— 2. Inspection

TEST ITEM

Instruction: On the line to the left of each term in Column A, write the letter of the statement in Column B that matches the term.

a. Use of the sense of touch to feel or press upon parts of the body.

b. The striking of an area of the body with fingers or instruments and listening to sounds produced.

BEHAVIORAL OBJECTIVE	TEST ITEM
— 3. Palpation	c. Use of the sense of hearing to interpret sounds produced within the body.
— 4. Auscultation	d. Visual examination for detection of features or qualities perceptible to the eye.
	e. The act of perceiving what is detected by the senses.

This format is a useful method of testing recall. It requires attention to details in construction so that the match between the two columns is unambiguous but not obvious.

Essay Question

The essay question, particularly beyond the knowledge level of the cognitive domain, not only tests the student's information about the subject matter but his/her ability to communicate ideas in a logical and coherent manner. It is used for all levels of the cognitive domain taxonomy, with the task called for in the question being the critical determinant of the level of cognition sought. The tasks signified for each level are stated similarly to the following.

Knowledge	How many, when, where, what name, list, define
Comprehension	Give illustrations, describe, explain, predict
Application	Give underlying principles, generalize, relate
Analysis	Analyze a problem, analyze data, compare, contrast, deduce
Synthesis	Formulate a new plan, design an approach, or write a perspective of an issue using relevant theories or concepts
Evaluation	Examine conclusions, judge accuracy, validity, reliability

The essay question, especially an open-ended one, is also useful in assessing development in the affective domain, especially at valuing or conceptualization levels. If an opinion is called for, the essay question is used only for formative evaluation, and the results cannot be graded. If, however, the cognitive base of the learner's opinion is requested, one may use the essay question in summative evaluation and translate the results into a grade. The opinion offered cannot be graded, but the logic of the rationale can be.

GENERAL PRINCIPLES OF CONSTRUCTION

1. The question should be constructed carefully so that the nature of the task is clearly stated. (The word discuss, used without a modifying phrase for direction, should be avoided, for it is too general a concept and does not give sufficient guidelines to the learner.)
2. The question should be constructed carefully so that exact limits of areas are clearly defined, i.e., a concept such as "care of the cardiac patient" is complicated and multidimensional. The student needs to know the focus of deliberations intended for the question, such as: psychosocial, pathophysiological, or economic dimensions. More than one dimension can be included in the question as long as the student knows the boundaries.
3. The desired outcome of the area tested should be set up as a basis for grading.
4. The student must know the basis of evaluation, especially where grading is to follow the evaluation. The basis might include:
   a. Evidence of meeting intended behaviors
   b. Evidence of the ability to select, organize, and present material in a coherent manner

Questions arise as to the appropriateness of evaluating grammar and spelling. If the essay question is a part of the in-class examination, the grammar and spelling should be evaluated but not graded, unless inaccuracies interfere with a coherent presentation. In an out-of-class examination, however, where the student has access to references, spelling and grammar should be considered legitimate competencies in communicating ideas.

ILLUSTRATIONS OF TYPES OF ESSAY QUESTIONS

BEHAVIORAL OBJECTIVES	TEST ITEM

Knowledge Level

C1.12   Recalls factors that influence man's ability to adapt.   List five factors that have an influence on man's capacity to adapt.

BEHAVIORAL OBJECTIVES	TEST ITEM
C1.23 Names, in order, the stages of the grief process.	List, in order, the stages of the grief process.

Comprehension Level

C2.1 Illustrates the stress-adaptation phenomenon.	Cite an example of a patient in stress and the adaptive response exhibited.
C2.2 Distinguishes between the behavior of integrity and that of despair in the elderly person.	Describe the behavior of the elderly person with a sense of integrity as it contrasts with that of the elderly person with a sense of despair.
C2.3 Makes inferences about the effect of air pollution on individuals with limited pulmonary function.	Predict the effects of smog on health of a person with emphysema.

Application Level

C3.0 Applies Erikson's crisis theory to the selection of appropriate nursing intervention.	Relate Erikson's crisis theory to the determination of the type of nursing intervention you would use in meeting the needs of parents with an acutely ill child.

Analysis Level

C4.1 Identifies assumptions underlying proposals for national health insurance.	Analyze one of the proposals for national health insurance and identify the assumptions underlying the major points in the plan.
C4.2 Analyzes the relationship between the adolescent developmental level and the societal pressures which have a bearing on the increase in venereal disease.	One county health department reported a marked increase in venereal disease among adolescents. How would you explain this phenomenon from the perspective of the relationship between the adolescent's developmental level and the pressures of society?
C4.3 Analyzes the form and pattern of a literary piece of work relevant to nursing.	Deduce the purpose, perspective, and feelings of the author in the book, *I Never Promised You a Rose Garden.*

BEHAVIORAL OBJECTIVES	TEST ITEM

Synthesis Level

C5.1   Writes an essay presenting a position on a health care issue.

Write an essay in which you present your reaction to the statement: Health is a human right.

C5.2   Proposes a plan of action for solving a problem within a health agency.

Write up a plan for combating institutional racism within a health agency.

C5.3   Formulates a conceptual scheme for categorizing nurse-patient interactions.

Devise a conceptual scheme for categorizing nurse-patient interactions in a family practice outpatient setting.

Evaluation Level

C6.1   Makes judgments of a report of a nursing research project in terms of internal criteria.

Select a clinical nursing research report in *Nursing Research*. Evaluate the work in terms of internal criteria: logical accuracy, validity, reliability, precision of statements, logic of conclusions from data, and appropriate documentation.

C6.2   Evaluates a nursing research report in terms of external criteria.

Select a nursing research report from *Nursing Research*. Compare this report with another comparable report in the same area that is recognized as a valid and reliable study.

The following two examples suggest ways in which the essay form of question might be used to test in the affective domain:

A3.2   Examines various points of view on a controversial issue with the intent of declaring a position on it.

"Welfare patients admitted to a medical center hospital should expect to be used for medical research."
1. Identify two possible positions in regard to this statement.
2. Provide a rationale for each position.
3. Specify your stand on the issue inherent in this statement and support your choice.

BEHAVIORAL OBJECTIVES	TEST ITEM
A4.1 Forms judgments as to the constitutional rights of individuals admitted to a mental care facility.	Using the Bill of Rights as a framework for your thinking, describe the constitutional rights of a person admitted to a mental care facility.

One of the major limitations in the use of essay questions is that the sampling of content in a course is restricted. However, especially at the upper levels of the taxonomies, essay questions are particularly useful as out-of-class examinations. The questions used for testing at the synthesis and evaluation cognitive levels, presented as illustrations, are more suitable to out-of-class examinations because of their nature and scope. The questions illustrating evaluation in the affective domain may be used in either out-of-class or in-class situations.

PROBLEM-SOLVING EVALUATION

Problem-solving evaluation may be used as part of a pencil and paper test, or it may be used as an evaluation project for a group of students. In the latter instance, members of the group discuss the questions and present results of their deliberations in writing or orally to the rest of the class.

The use of problem-solving situations is designed to assess the student's ability for critical thinking. The student is presented with a written description of a nursing problem situation and is then asked to respond to questions relative to the situation. The format of questions used in a situation may vary. One format, such as multiple recognition, may be used for all questions or a variety of test item forms, such as multiple recognition, essay, and alternate response may be used for testing.

Three types of test exercises are usually associated with this classification of evaluation—situation, critical incident, and decision making. Problem situations expressed in any of these three types often test more than one behavioral objective per situation and may be used with any level of the cognitive and affective domains.

GENERAL PRINCIPLES OF CONSTRUCTION

1. The problem-solving situation should be geared to the learner's knowledge and experience.
2. Information about the incident or situation should be sufficient to assure clarity in the presentation.

3. The situation must be reasonable in length so that the learner is not required to devote a long period of time reading and rereading the description.
4. The critical incident needs to be sharply presented with no extraneous material included.
5. Questions posed must be related directly to the data incorporated in the descriptions.

Situation

The situation test, based on the field theory of learning, describes a situation pertinent to nursing which incorporates all data significant to understanding the nature of the problem. Questions directed to this form relate to nursing actions, to the theoretical basis for nursing practice, or to the application of theory to nursing actions, as indicated in the situation.

ILLUSTRATIONS

ILLUSTRATION I
BEHAVIORAL OBJECTIVES

A3.1   Expresses own feelings about ways individuals respond to stress.

C4.1   Deduces stress factors in a patient-family situation.

C3.0   Applies stress adaptation theory to a patient's situation.

INSTRUCTIONS

Read the following situation and then answer the questions.

SITUATION

Ms. J, a 20-year-old mother of three children, ranging in age from six months to three years, lives with her mother and younger brother in a three room tenement in the ghetto area of the city. Never married, Ms. J has been receiving assistance from Aid to Dependent Children since the birth of her first child.

During last evening, Ms. J was brought to the emergency ward of the hospital in acute distress from heroin overdose. She is now a patient in the hospital ward and you have been assigned to provide her with nursing care.

QUESTIONS

1. What are your feelings about Ms. J as you prepare to plan her care?
2. What stressors do you identify in her life situation as described here?
3. Explain the dynamics of this patient-family situation on the basis of the stress-adaptation theory.
4. What is your opinion about the way Ms. J is handling her stressors?

ILLUSTRATION II
BEHAVIORAL OBJECTIVES

C4.2   Relates patient's reaction to impending death to the stage in the grief process being experienced.

C4.2   Responds to patient's concerns consistent with his reaction to impending death.

A4.1   Explores own values about death as they relate to the variables of age and cause of death.

INSTRUCTIONS

Read the following situation and then answer the questions according to the stated directions.

SITUATION

John, a 16-year-old, has leukemia and knows it. Readmitted to the hospital for the third time, now in critical condition, he says to the nurse, "It is good I had to come this time during summer vacation, so I am not going to waste any more time from school. You know, I'll graduate from high school in one year and I want to keep my A average to go straight to college. In this way it will not take me more than four years to become a lawyer since the doctors told me it doesn't look too good for me."

QUESTIONS

1. John's comments suggest that he is in the _____ stage of the grief process.

2. The mechanism by which John is handling the stress of dying is called _____.

Circle the letter that appears in front of the *one* statement that completes correctly the statement in questions 3 and 4.

3. If you were the nurse, your interpretation of John's statement would be:
   a. John has not understood the doctor's explanation about the fatal prognosis of his disease.
   b. John acts as a typical adolescent who is trying to impress you with his scholastic performance.
   c. John knows about his prognosis, but denies it.
   d. John knows about his prognosis, but bargains for the time left.

4. To help John progress through the grief process, the best response you could make to his comment would be:
   a. "Congratulations, John, I am glad to know that you are a good student."
   b. "Does it bother you that this disease might interfere with your studies, John?"
   c. "You are right, John, so you will be in good shape when school starts in September."
   d. "Don't worry about school now, John. The important thing is that you will be feeling better."

Circle the "A" before the following statements with which you agree; circle the "D" before the following statements with which you disagree; and circle the "U" before the following statements about which you are uncertain. Support your choice in the space provided.

5. A. U. D.   John's death from leukemia is more tragic than it would have been if his death occurred on the battlefield.

6. A. U. D.   It is more tragic for John to die of leukemia than for a man of 60 to die from the same disease.

7. A. U. D.   John's comments suggest he is making an appropriate adaptation to the stress caused by his impending death.

Critical Incident

Critical incident is the second form of evaluation suggested under the rubric of problem solving. It is a description of an event in which data are limited to factors that have a direct bearing on the event itself. Questions in this area generally relate to a nursing judgment and/or actions such as: assessment, interpretation of data, prediction of consequences, formulation of hypotheses, suggestions for intervention, or determination of criteria for evaluation.

ILLUSTRATIONS

ILLUSTRATION I
BEHAVIORAL OBJECTIVE

C2.2   Determine types of data appropriate for a nursing decision.

INSTRUCTIONS

Read the incident below and respond to the question.

CRITICAL INCIDENT

A nurse enters the room of a 45-year-old male to take his blood pressure as ordered q4h. She finds that the reading is 80/50, a drop from 100/80 at the reading four hours ago.

QUESTION

What questions should the nurse raise to focus the data collection necessary for determining the decision for action?

ILLUSTRATION II
BEHAVIORAL OBJECTIVES

A3.1   Examines own feelings about the elderly person's need to live a meaningful life.

C3.0   Uses relevant theories in interpreting the dynamics in a critical incident.

INSTRUCTIONS

Read the incident below and respond to the questions.

CRITICAL INCIDENT

Three months after the death of his wife of 52 years, you see Mr. A, an 81-year-old man, walking down the street holding hands with a female contemporary. They are laughing and appear happy.

QUESTIONS

1. What would be your initial reaction upon seeing Mr. A and his friend? Why do you react in this manner?
2. How does Mr. A's behavior relate to the Erikson concept of the age of integrity?
3. Relate your concept of human sexuality to the interaction between Mr. A and his friend.
4. How do you really feel about Mr. A's behavior?

Decision-Making

This form of question provides a description of a nursing action that involves a nursing decision. Three approaches to decision-making exercises may be used:

1. Describe a situation up to a point of decision. Ask the student to make the decision indicated and provide a rationale for the choice.
2. Describe a situation, including the decision. Ask the student to state agreement or disagreement with the decision and support response.
3. Describe the situation, including the decision. Ask the student if the information provided is sufficient for a decision. If the response is in the negative ask the student to indicate what other information is indicated.

(In some instances 2 and 3 are combined.)

The decision-making process involves identifying clues indicating that a decision is necessary, assessing the situation, selecting alternatives for action considering consequences of each action, establishing priority of choices, and evaluating the outcomes. This type of evaluation is especially important in helping the student develop divergent thinking ability, the process by which the student arrives at several alternative solutions. It is the requirement of the student's recognition of alternatives and the selection of the best of the alternatives that makes this type of test situation a particularly valuable evaluation strategy for determining the student's critical thinking competency.

ILLUSTRATIONS

ILLUSTRATION I
BEHAVIORAL OBJECTIVE

C3.0   Uses decision-making process in meeting the expressed needs of an individual.

INSTRUCTIONS

Read the situation below and respond to the questions.

DECISION-MAKING INCIDENT

Mr. P, a forty-eight-year-old college professor, has inoperable cancer. No one has informed him of his diagnosis. One morning while you are providing care to him he states, "I wish someone would tell me what is wrong with me." You feel that his statement calls for a decision for action.

QUESTIONS

1. What clue(s) in the situation have convinced you that a decision is indicated?
2. What is your assessment of Mr. P's situation?
3. Identify three alternative courses of action that could be taken.
4. Describe the possible consequences of each course of action.
5. What decision would you select? Support your choice of decision.

ILLUSTRATION II
BEHAVIORAL OBJECTIVE

C4.2   Analyzes a decision for a nursing action from the perspective of the decision-making process.

INSTRUCTIONS

Read the situation below and respond to the questions accordingly.

DECISION-MAKING INCIDENT

A senior nursing student in a public health experience made a visit with the instructor. The purpose of the visit was the health supervision of a premature male infant now nine months old. It is the practice of the health department to follow premature infants for one year.

Mrs. Brown greeted the student warmly, stating that she was glad for the visit because her son, John, seemed to be ailing. She stated, "He must have broken out during the night. He wasn't sick yesterday, why we even visited my next door neighbor. She's pretty excited because she thinks she's pregnant. She missed two periods."

The student examined the baby and noted a generalized rash and enlarged cervical nodes. Suspecting rubella, the student shared her findings with Mrs. Brown. She urged Mrs. Brown to take John to the physician for diagnosis and any necessary treatment.

QUESTIONS

1. What is the decision for action the nursing student made?
   Do you agree with it? Yes _____ No _____
2. Are the data sufficient for you as the nurse in this situation to make a decision?
   Yes _____ No _____
   If no, what other data would you need?
3. Analyze this situation in terms of each step of the decision-making process.
4. What decision would you make if you were the nursing student in this situation? Support your choice.

Problem-solving situations are designed to test levels of cognitive ability beyond the skill of recall. Nursing, as a practice discipline, uses knowledge. Therefore, evaluation procedures that call upon students to demonstrate competency in using knowledge are of particular significance. Problem-solving test strategies provide data that help to identify the theoretical base of the learner's actions, as distinct from intuition or imitation. These test situations also help both the learner and teacher to be aware of values the learner holds, and to assess these values as to their appropriateness to a practitioner in a helping profession.

MULTIMEDIA

The use of multimedia in educational programs has increased markedly during the past decade, but its use in evaluation has been limited. Multimedia increase the variety of senses, such as hearing, touching, and seeing images, used by the student during an evaluation experience. The increased sensory stimulation adds more depth in a test situation and increases the scope of evaluation. Multimedia are especially amenable to simulation testing.

In previous illustrations of problem-solving situations, there was sole reliance on the written word. If visual imagery and tonal qualities were added to the situations so that the learner could see the participants engaged in action and hear their conversations, then the whole evaluation experience would take on more dynamic dimensions and the student could become more involved in the process. If the student had been able to see Mr. A and his female companion, this direct contact may have elicited a more accurate response than would be possible simply as a result of reading about the incident.

Multimedia may be used with other forms of evaluation. Questions may be posed in any of the formats previously discussed in this chapter. They may be used in in-class situations; although they are particularly effective for out-of-class exercises, especially where students have access to a learning laboratory. Many types of hardware may be used for projecting the test situations. The following suggestions are made for consideration in the use of films, videotapes, tapes, slides, and pictures.

Films provide for visual and, in most cases, auditory stimulation. Added stimuli facilitate testing of students' problem-solving abilities and help in determining the values and beliefs upon which students base their actions. A film situation may depict events such as nursing actions; patient behavior; individual, family, or group responses to phenomena in a setting; or action within an environment. They are particularly useful in critical-incident testing and decision-making testing.

Videotapes are a more recent development in the evaluation field. They provide for visual and auditory stimulation and have a start-stop capability. Their use is similar to the use of films, except in instances where videotapes are made of the learner in a practice situation. In this instance, videotapes are an effective means of formative evaluation, for the learner and the teacher (and in some instances other learners) have the opportunity to appraise the learner's practice and analyze it critically.

Tape recording is a current development in our society and adds an auditory dimension to the evaluation strategy. It can be used with illustrations of music, poetry, literature reading, verbal interactions among or between individuals in group work, and various sounds, such as heart and lung. The tape recording approach may be used to assess a student's competency in interpreting or analyzing interviews, the patient-nurse teaching situations, the group process, or an individual's expression of ideas, beliefs, or values. Now that nurses are becoming more involved in physical assessment skills, evaluation of the learner's ability to discriminate body sounds may be assisted by the tape recording strategy.

When tapes are used in conjunction with film strips or slides, visual stimulation is added and topics used for evaluation can be extended to problem-solving situations, as described for films.

Slides and pictures provide for visual imagery. They may be used in attitude testing, as, for example, when a student is requested to interpret the meaning of the scene depicted. They may also serve as an important means of assessing the student's ability to make critical judgments relative to the "rightness" or "wrongness" of some aspect portrayed. This type of judgment may relate to such images as the method of holding a baby, methods for positioning patients, the posture of a nurse while carrying out a specific action, or the characteristics of an environment. Slide series may represent steps in a process that may be interpreted or critically analyzed by the learner.

GENERAL PRINCIPLES OF CONSTRUCTION

1. Selection of the appropriate multimedia device must be determined by the behavioral objective.
2. Unless the learner has access to the equipment used for the test situation for repeated viewing or listening, the situation for the test should be short enough (about 1-3 minutes) for the student to remember.
3. Behaviors to be evaluated as well as the test questions should be presented to the student before the test situation is turned on so that the student will be able to focus attention on significant aspects.
4. Questions can only relate to the events depicted in the situation.
5. When visual imagery is used in class situations, all students must have a clear and unobstructed view.

ILLUSTRATIONS

ILLUSTRATION OF TAPE RECORDING
BEHAVIORAL OBJECTIVE

C4.1   Differentiates the sounds elicited when percussion technique is used.

INSTRUCTIONS

Listen to the tape recording, "Sounds in Percussion", and answer the following questions.

QUESTIONS

1. Identify the different percussion sounds recorded on the tape.
2. Describe the differentiating characteristics of each sound.
3. Identify a location in the body where each type of sound may be heard.

ILLUSTRATION OF SLIDES AND TAPE RECORDING
BEHAVIORAL OBJECTIVES

C2.2   Distinguishes the stereotyped comments made by the nurse.

C3.0   Chooses two alternative approaches the nurse could have used in greeting the patient.

C2.1   Cites examples of own stereotyped responses in handling anxiety.

INSTRUCTIONS

View the single-concept slide series and listen to the accompanying tape for "Interactions for Study" and respond to the questions accordingly.

(This vignette depicts a nurse conversing with a patient who has had a C.V.A. While exercising the patient's affected arm, the nurse responds to the patient's expressed concerns in a trite and nonlistening manner.)

QUESTIONS

1. Identify at least two stereotypic comments made by the nurse during this interaction.
2. Write two alternate approaches the nurse could use to convey her interest and concern for how Mrs. Bolin is feeling. Explain how the approaches you suggest differ from those in the filmstrip.
3. Describe an incident in which you have felt anxious while interacting with a patient. What stereotypic responses did you give in that situation?

ILLUSTRATION OF THE USE OF A FILM

BEHAVIORAL OBJECTIVE

C4.1   Identifies the nursing functions of the clinic nurse in meeting the needs of the pregnant woman.

INSTRUCTIONS

View the section of the film, *A World of Contrasts: A Time of Hope,* which portrays the visit of a pregnant woman to the clinic, and then respond to the questions.

(This film has six separate episodes, each portraying a concept of public health nursing. The episode used for this testing shows primarily a young pregnant woman and a clinic nurse in interaction, although there are a few views of a parent-teaching class.)

QUESTIONS

In the film, a pregnant woman comes to the clinic for prenatal care.
1. What nursing functions are identified as the responsibility of the nurse in this situation?
2. Are you satisfied that the functions identified are compatible with the concept of primary-care nursing?

Yes _____ No _____

If not, what changes or additions would you suggest based on the concept of primary-care nursing in this type of health care setting?

Programmed and computer assisted instruction have a built-in evaluation process. Both incorporate the principle of feedback and direct the learner forward in the learning exercise when a question is answered correctly. The evaluation strategy is programmed and thus not subject to development or modification by a particular teacher or learner.

Whether designed for a printed page or for a machine and whether developed in a linear or branching style, the programs are based on the behavioristic concept of reinforcement. This feedback approach is relevant to formative evaluation for it provides the teacher and learner with clues as to areas of learning difficulty in the attainment of the stated behavioral objectives.

Multimedia add sensory dimensions to the evaluation process and have greater potential for involving the learner who is called upon more and more to respond to a greater variety of sensory stimuli.

PAPERS AND OTHER WRITTEN ASSIGNMENTS

Written work provides teachers with an excellent opportunity to assess the student's ability relative to the thinking process, the communication of ideas, and the values and beliefs operant. (Some of the written work is more relevant to clinical practice and will be discussed in the following chapter.) Critical analysis of readings, phenomena or situations, essays, defense of positions on issues, and reports of studies can follow the patterns previously illustrated. Many of the suggestions for questions stated in the essay section are particularly pertinent. Further illustrative examples will not be given, but some general principles are offered.

GENERAL PRINCIPLES

1. The behavioral objective(s) for the assignment must be stated clearly.
2. Instructions must be stated clearly and understood by the learner.
3. Provision should be made for individual guidance as the need is indicated, so that the student can aspire to mastery.
4. Learners should be notified of standards for evaluation and the basis for grading.
5. Faculty should support creative approaches to meeting objectives.
6. Written work deviating from the prescribed format should be assessed in terms of its response to the objectives, not its adherence to an expected form.

GROUP PROJECTS

Evaluation of individual performance based on specific, individual strategies causes less concern for teachers than evaluation of an individual in a group activity. The question arises as to whether or not all individuals in a group should receive the same evaluation and perhaps the same grade. Questions relate to equity in the quality of each member's participation. If there is no equity, the teacher must decide what measures are just and fair for discriminating differences. Evaluation of a group project should provide opportunity for assessing the group as a whole as well as individual performance within the group.

GENERAL PRINCIPLES

1. As with any evaluation procedure, group activities are directed toward achieving behavioral objectives on which the group will be evaluated.
2. Faculty and students participate in determining behaviors that will be used to evaluate the group.
3. Behaviors include those appropriate to the substance of the report as well as to standards of communication.
4. The evaluation also provides for comments that evidence discrimination among the participants' attainment of the behaviors.
5. There must be provision for process as well as outcome evaluation.
6. Group members evaluate each other's participation in the group.
7. When group presentation is given before a class or a similar group, all viewers of the presentation participate in the evaluation.
8. When group presentation is given before a class or a similar group, the evaluation form is completed immediately after the presentation while the perception of the process is clear in the mind of the evaluators.

ILLUSTRATION—GROUP PRESENTATION BEFORE A CLASS

Figure 8-1 illustrates a form that was used to evaluate the performance of a group of students who presented a project for the course *Perspectives in Nursing*. The content behaviors are those designed for the project. This form, developed by students and faculty, was completed by participants in the group as well as by members of the class, and was submitted at the conclusion of each group's presentation. Data were analyzed and a profile for each group was determined as well as a content analysis on items 3 and 4.

Figure 8-2 shows the second evaluation form used in the project. As with the previous form, this was developed jointly by faculty and students, and each participant in the presenting group completed a self-evaluation and also evaluated colleagues in the group. The focus was to assist the assessment of

Perspectives in Nursing

EVALUATION OF GROUP PROJECT

Topic:
Date:
Participants:

Behavioral objectives relative to the presentation of the Task Force reports are listed below. Opposite each behavioral objective is a scale representing the degrees of attainment. *Circle the number* on the scale which you feel best represents the group's attainment of the objective.

I. *Content*
    1. Defines the issue.   (not attained) 1 2 3 4 5 6 (attained)

    2. Describes the present state of   .   (not attained) 1 2 3 4 5 6 (attained)
        the issue including supportive
        and constraining factors.

    3. Discriminates elements which   (not attained) 1 2 3 4 5 6 (attained)
        make it an issue.

    4. Describes the meaning of the   (not attained) 1 2 3 4 5 6 (attained)
        issue to nursing and to society.

    5. Deduces the origin of the is-   (not attained) 1 2 3 4 5 6 (attained)
        sue.

    6. Describes the status of the   (not attained) 1 2 3 4 5 6 (attained)
        issue within the context of soc-
        iety at particular periods of
        time.

    7. Identifies role of particular in-   (not attained) 1 2 3 4 5 6 (attained)
        dividuals who had a significant
        impact on the issue through-
        out its course.

    8. Predicts the state of the issue   (not attained) 1 2 3 4 5 6 (attained)
        in the future.

    9. Presents a hypothesis for the   (not attained) 1 2 3 4 5 6 (attained)
        future.

    10. Provides   rationale   for   (not attained) 1 2 3 4 5 6 (attained)
        hypothesis.

    11. Identifies changes necessary   (not attained) 1 2 3 4 5 6 (attained)
        for the future prediction.

Fig. 8-1. Sample Form for Evaluation of Group Project.

II. *Method of Presentation*
1. Organizes presentation in a   (not attained) 1 2 3 4 5 6 (attained)
clear, logical manner.

2. Communicates ideas clearly.   (not attained) 1 2 3 4 5 6 (attained)

3. Evidences continuity among   (not attained) 1 2 3 4 5 6 (attained)
presenters.

4. Makes provisions for discus-   (not attained) 1 2 3 4 5 6 (attained)
sion by class members.

5. Responds to questions in a   (not attained) 1 2 3 4 5 6 (attained)
knowledgeable manner.

6. Shows originality in the pre-   (not attained) 1 2 3 4 5 6 (attained)
sentation.

III. *General Comments*

IV. *Comments Regarding Specific Participants*

Fig. 8-1. *(cont.)*

Perspectives in Nursing

EVALUATION OF INDIVIDUAL PARTICIPATION

Name of Participant:

Topic of Group:

Rate each of the five behaviors listed below, circle the appropriate numbers, and support your position in the space provided.

1. Assumes responsibility for own   (Little) 1 2 3 4 5 6 7 (Much)
share of the work.
COMMENT:

2. Helps rest of the group in getting   (Little) 1 2 3 4 5 6 7 (Much)
resources.
COMMENT:

Fig. 8-2. Sample Form for Evaluation of Individual Participation.

3. Willingly shares ideas with col-   (Little) 1 2 3 4 5 6 7 (Much)
    leagues.
    COMMENT:

4. Brings new ideas to the group.   (Little) 1 2 3 4 5 6 7 (Much)
    COMMENT:

5. Shares leadership, responsibility.   (Little) 1 2 3 4 5 6 7 (Much)
    COMMENT:

6. Other comments.

Fig. 8-2.   (cont.)

each member as to performance during the developmental process of the
project. Data were analyzed and a profile made for each of the participants.

Both of these strategies enabled evaluation of the total group presentation
as well as the participation of each member.

ILLUSTRATION—SEMINAR

In a seminar, another group activity, the issues of evaluation are different
from the group project described above. The student participates as a leader
and as a contributing member at various times throughout the seminar.

Figure 8-3 is an illustration of the behaviors identified by a group of
graduate students in a seminar course. Each member evaluated every other
member of the group. The procedure identifies four major variables—
leadership role in the seminar, quality of the content of the presentation,
quality of the presentation, and the participant role. Students identified
behaviors expected under each heading and used them to write a descriptive
evaluation of each other at the end of the course. It might be noted that the
same form was used to evaluate the faculty member, who was considered a
seminar member and responsible for presenting one of the seminars. The
evaluations were summarized for each student.

Evaluation of group projects must provide opportunity to gather data on
individual as well as on group performance. This involves student-teacher
participation in determining behaviors as well as in the process itself. In
addition to obtaining a data base for evaluative judgment, this approach also
enables the student to gain experience in self-evaluation and in the evaluation of others.

Seminar in Nursing Education

EVALUATIONS

Name: SEMINAR Member:

1. Leadership Role in Seminar
   Shares leadership responsibility with colleagues.
   Modifies plan when indicated on the basis of analysis of group dynamics.
   Supports participants in their efforts to be active in the group process.
   Provides for freedom of thought and expression of all participants.
   Helps the group synthesize ideas presented.

2. Quality of Content of Presentation
   Prepares objectives which encourage an analytic approach.
   Proposes readings which are relevant to the objectives.
   Develops content on an appropriate theoretical basis.
   Relates content to stated objectives.
   Analyzes issues in terms of their relationship to society, the profession, and self.
   Analyzes issues in terms of past, present, and future dimensions.

3. Quality of Presentation
   Organizes material in a clear manner.
   Explains material in a clear, comprehensive manner.
   Utilizes methods appropriate to presentation.
   Plans presentation so as to allow for group participation.
   Clarifies points when indicated.

4. Participant Role in Seminar
   Supports viewpoints with rationale.
   Contributes to the discussion in a scholarly fashion.
   Willingly shares ideas and feelings with colleagues.
   Respects right of all individuals to agree/disagree with one's opinion.
   Is able to agree/disagree with idea without attacking individual.
   Uses intellectual discipline in handling disagrekement.
   Analyzes effect of self on group process.

Figure 8-3. Sample Form for Seminar Evaluation.

SUMMARY

There is a direct relationship between the *what* and the *how* of evaluation. Evaluation strategies must be appropriate to specified behavior.

In any educational endeavor, it is important that a variety of strategies be prepared to meet the individual needs of learners and the particular nature of the situation. Efforts must be made to direct evaluation at the cognitive level beyond that of recall, for nurses must be able to demonstrate competency in their use of knowledge in a variety of circumstances. Evaluation must also include strategies for determining the affective as well as the cognitive level of development, for values are determinants of behavior.

Use of the taxonomies in defining expected behavior is helpful in stating the level desired. It is essential, however, that the evaluation procedure be designed in such a way as to be compatible with the specified behavior. Various strategies include: paper and pencil tests (alternate response, multiple recognition, completion, matching, and essay); problem solving (situation, critical incident, and decision making); multimedia (films, videotapes, tape recordings, slides, pictures); papers and other written work; and group projects.

REFERENCE

1. Hoffman B. Tyranny of Testing. New York: Crowell-Collier Press, 1962, pp. 89–101.

RECOMMENDED READINGS

Barr, D.: A Note on the Technology of Cynicism. Columbia University Forum 6:33, 1963.

Evaluation of Nursing Educational Achievement. Report of CENTO Workshop, Ankara, Turkey, 1973

Friedenberg, E. The Real Functions of Educational Testing. *Change* 2:43, 1970.

Harmin, M., Kirschenbaum, H. & Simon, S. Clarifying Values through Subject Matter. Minneapolis: Winston Press, 1973.

Heidgerken, L. Teaching and Learning in Schools of Nursing. Philadelphia:Lippincott, 1965.

Karmel Louis, J. and Karmel, M.O. Measurement and Evaluation in the Schools, (2nd ed.). New York:Macmillan, 1978.

Quiring, J. D. Utilizing Questioning Strategies in Nursing Education. J Nurs Educ, 12:21, 1973.

Robbins, Eric, Examining Examinations, *Nursing Times*, a weekly series presented in 8 parts, beginning in Oct. 16, 1975 publication.

Scholdra, J. D., Quiring J. D.: The Level of Questions Posed by Nursing Education. J Nurs Educ, 12:15, 1973.

Shields, M. R.: The Construction and Use of Teacher-Made Tests. New York:National League for Nursing, 1965.

Smeltzer, C. H. Psychological Evaluations in Nursing Education. New York:Macmillan, 1965.

Steele, S. Educational Evaluation in Nursing, Thorofare, N.J.:Charles Slack, 1978.

9 Test Construction

What will be on the test? Will we be responsible for this on our final? What will the exam cover? Do these questions sound familiar? How often do faculty hear students raise these questions before examination time? Why are these questions being raised? What are students really saying?

The students' questions are really symptomatic of a serious malady of the testing process and its relationship to the total educational endeavor.

TESTING PROCESS

Eble[1] (1976) suggests that there are three crucial questions faculty must ask relative to the testing of students: (1) Why am I testing? (2) How am I testing? (3) What results am I getting?

Why Am I Testing?

Why am I testing? The questions used to introduce this chapter should provide some clue to the students' perceptions of why they are being tested. The students' questions arise out of a need to survive and to achieve an acceptable grade since most testing generates grades. The concept of acceptable grade varies among students; from the highly competitive achiever who must attain the highest grade to the individual who must achieve at least the minimum passing level. Regardless of the individual student's definition of acceptable grade, the reality of the grade becomes a prime motivation as the test situation approaches. Recognizing that docility and conformity are important strategies for survival, the student feels the need to be able to respond to the test according to the wishes of the teacher. The student's perception of what is worth knowing as a result of the learning experience is often that which will be on the test.

How do teachers answer the question, *Why am I testing?* How compatible are their perceptions of the purpose of testing with those of the student? Is there not a dimension of the teacher's perception which may be a major contributing factor to the student's perception of testing and the anxiety associated with the survival need? Do teachers see testing as a strategy for maintaining control of the learning situation? The warning to the student, "You had better know this material for it will be on the test," is not an infrequent occurrence, especially if a student elects to be absent from the classroom session. One cannot deny the power disparity between student and faculty. The way the teacher uses that power is a major factor in the student's perception of the testing process.

This introduction to the testing process is a negative one, yet it does represent reality in most situations. Testing makes participants uncomfortable. Teachers themselves often do not like tests because they may impinge on an amicable relationship with students. On the other hand, they may like tests because they can be used to control the students' learning. Students dislike tests because they perceive them as traps that foster the need for compliance with what the teacher wants. Experience with unannounced quizzes, unexpected material being tested, and emphasis on testing minutiae all contribute to the student's perception of testing as a checking process or a battle of wits.

But need tests be so threatening and destructive to the pursuit of learning? Is there not a human need "to know what I know?" How many individuals enjoy doing crossword puzzles, answering quizzes that appear in popular magazines, or vicariously responding to questions on television programs? It is this basic need *to know what I know* that is so destroyed by our present education practices. In the educational system, the need to know is often not for the pure joy and satisfaction of the pursuit of self-knowledge, but rather for survival.

Testing is important and has a significant role in the educational process. Its feedback provides much data which have the potential for contributing to the growth of the student and teacher, as well as the development of the course or program. The diagnostic function of a test is most significant, yet it is seldom used. Indeed the diagnostic potential is ignored in courses that primarily emphasize the final examination, for by the time the test is given, the student's exposure to learning opportunities to redress the difficulties have ceased.

Tests can and should be used for both formative and summative evaluation purposes. It is essential that the teacher clearly define which of these purposes is basic to the particular test. One must remember that summative evaluation is also diagnostic, but the diagnosis is concerned with future learning, not the current one in which the student has been participating.

Used within a systematic formative and summative evaluation protocol, testing is most important in helping the student know what knowledge has been acquired and where there has been failure in understanding or in achieving competency. The teacher in such a process is able to determine the degree to which the objectives are achieved. The effectiveness of the teaching is also revealed since students indicate what they have learned or what they have not learned or understood.

How Am I Testing?

The question, How am I testing?, addresses two factors: the substance of the test and the testing strategies employed.

The substance of tests is often a source of great irritation and mistrust for students. One hears many complaints about the testing of trivia. Brunner (1963) addresses the issue of trivia testing as he talks about the structure of a discipline in his book, *Process of Education*. His comment regarding material worth knowing is paraphrased for nursing education.[2] "Whether when fully developed as practitioners the subject or material is worth a graduate nurse's knowing and whether having known it as a student makes a person a better graduate nurse." Brunner challenges the educator to sort out the essentials from the trivia in teaching. Testing should be directed toward the essentials.

How are these essentials identified for both the teacher and the learner? The statement of behavioral objectives clearly denotes the subject matter to be learned and the behavior the student is expected to achieve in relation to this subject matter. Course unit examinations and quizzes must be based on predetermined objectives so that both teacher and learner know the focus of the evaluation. The student's need to outguess what the teacher wants is incompatible with sound testing principles. The process for selecting testable content from the objectives is described later in this chapter.

The search for objective examinations is in vain, although individuals do often refer to *objective examinations*. The latter suggests certain formats that are readily scored and limit the options the responder has in answering the questions. The subjective element is inherent in their very choice and, except for those addressed to known facts, the items often reflect the bias or the cultural values of the designers. The existence of the culturally biased test items which limit the use of many tests with certain populations is an established fact. The criterion of *fairness* is perhaps more realistic than a criterion of *objective*.

Regardless of the test format, fair questions can be developed which enable the student to discover what has been learned, not whether one has been successful in "beating the system." One aspect of fairness relates to the student's understanding of the behavior to be tested. An objective that charges the student to develop the ability to *analyze* a phenomenon and demonstrate that competency in an evaluation situation does not permit the teacher to evaluate the ability to *recall* five components of the phenomenon. In other words, the testing strategy used and the question asked must be compatible with the behavior stated in the objective. If the students know beforehand the nature of the subject matter and the behavior to be demonstrated, then the student can approach the testing situation with a considerable degree of confidence. The energy needed to psych out the teacher and to try to determine what the student is expected to know for the test is instead expended toward needs relative to achievement on the test. The student has a right to know what is expected on any test. There is no room in the testing process for the unexpected or unanticipated. Fairness demands accountability on the part of both student and teacher.

The question, How am I testing?, suggests another area of concern to faculty. This concern relates to the format used by faculty. How much variety in test design appears in the tests offered? Evidence suggests that faculty tend to get into a rut with many of these testing practices. They use the same general format each time. The end result is a test situation that is boring; teachers are bored and students are bored. There is no excitement, but only boredom resulting from predictability and redundancy.

What Results Am I Getting?

The third question, What results am I getting?, is closely allied to the two preceding questions. The expectation of results is determined by the reason for testing and the process of testing. Unfortunately, some faculty look at testing as a form of triage—a way of separating out the "smart ones" from the "poor ones" and the "in-betweens." For some, the results often confirm prejudgments and function as a self-fulfilling prophecy. However, for most faculty, the results serve the function of diagnostic feedback mentioned earlier. The results not only provide data about the performance of individual students, but they provide the teacher with some awareness of a class norm. Plans for assessing the results need to be carefully designed prior to the examination following the practice done with all other aspects of the test development.

TEST DEVELOPMENT

Although it is acknowledged that in our present educational society testing is often perceived as a threat to the ego and a menace to self development, it is also acknowledged that testing has a significant role in our educational process. The menace is not from testing itself, but rather from the misuse of the process. As an anology, automobiles are important in our life style. They are not a menace in themselves, but rather become a menace as they are misused. The goal is to develop and use tests to serve as a facilitating process in nursing education, not as a deterrent.

Purpose

Two major approaches to testing the achievement of the student are available, and it is essential that the teacher determine which approach will be used in the examination being prepared. The development of test items and the interpretation of results are dependent upon this choice.

A *norm-referenced test* is developed with the intent of comparing a student's achievement in relation to that of the student's classmates or peer group. A relative standard is used in interpreting the results—the standard being the average performance of a group. Test data are analyzed from the perspective of the normal curve. Standardized tests are the most common example of this approach to testing.

A *criterion-referenced test* is developed with the intent of comparing a student's achievement in relation to performance standards. An absolute standard is used in interpreting results—the standard being acceptably defined prior to the testing situation. This form of testing was developed as a result of the concept of mastery of learning and highlights the student's attainment of the objectives of a program in relation to specific criteria. It is the testing approach most applicable to most testing events within a nursing program, especially since competency is a critical outcome.

The planning for the testing program of each course must consider the purpose of the particular test. Is the test to provide data about the student's performance according to the absolute or the relative standard? Are the test results to be used primarily for formative or summative evaluation? Not all tests should be administered for the purpose of grading. Are the tests designed to determine student achievement in the cognitive and the affective domains, or is only one domain to be tested?

There are other reasons for testing than the primary one of determining competency. Some tests may be designed to discriminate types of competency among various classifications of learners. One faculty member decided that there was a time in the course when all students needed some sense of accomplishment; so he designed a test that all students could master. Sometimes a test will be administered to acquaint the student with a certain format of testing. There is in reality a state of being *test wise*, the situation where a test result may reflect more an individual's skill in test-taking than competency in the subject matter the test is designed to measure.

There are multiple purposes for testing. It is important that the test designer know the purpose(s) for the test being prepared and that the students are also clear as to the purpose. The purpose, however, must take into account the other types of evaluative data being collected on the student. Since all evaluation is designed to assess competency of the student, there must be a relationship among all data generated by the various strategies. A test by itself will not be sufficient as the only evaluative strategy.

Planning

The following scenario is seen all too frequently in schools of nursing as tests are prepared.

It is less than a week before the final examination is to be administered. In a small conference room in a school of nursing, four faculty can be observed around the table. On the table are some open textbooks, copies of previous examinations, and lecture notes. Conversation goes as follows: "Shall we ask them this in the exam?" "Was this covered in class?" "How about using this question again since everyone ought to know this?" "They were all supposed to read this chapter, let's ask a question from this chapter"–End of this scenario.

The scene, faculty preparing a final examination, now needs some analysis. How many errors are identifiable in this scene? Errors:

1. Time for planning was too close to examination.
2. Focus of the examination had no direction. It reflected a concept of teaching as telling and suggested a recall testing process.
3. No objectives for the course were evident to guide the test makers in the selection of content and testing strategy.
4. There was a suggestion of using this examination as a means of checking to see if students did their assignment.
5. The conversation evidenced the "they and us" syndrome. Students were never referred to as students, but always in the form of third person plural.

Unfortunately, the process of test development first presented is all too common. Test preparation is generally an "add on" activity with little evidence of careful planning, yet its use for influencing the life and careers of students is awesome. Planning for testing must be integrated into the total planning process of each course or unit. Not only the location of the testing within the course framework must be identified, but also the development of each test must be as carefully processed as is the content and all learning activities. In reality, the testing should be prepared before the course is even taught. If testing is used to determine the achievement of the student relative to the objective, then the testing can be developed once the objectives have been stated. Testing is not dependent upon what is covered in class.

Once rationale for the various testing periods within a course has been determined, it is essential that the time frame allocated to each testing period be designated. The time frame will be determined by the purpose and will have some influence on the sampling of behaviors to be tested and the strategies to be used.

The planning for the testing and the identification of its purpose within the total educational endeavor makes it imperative that appropriate tests be devised. Lenberg[3] (1978) suggests three concepts that are critical to the development of appropriate tests for performance evaluation. These three concepts, (1) content, (2) characteristics, (3) structure and process, provide a framework for test construction as well.

Selection of Content

Content relates to the subject matter of the test and the desired behavior the student is to exhibit. In written tests, the behavior is primarily cognitive. Affective behaviors can be tested at a lower level by suggesting a value preference behavior in response to a situation and at a higher level by requiring the student to respond cognitively to the rationale behind the behavior. The patterning behavior essential for validating true value commitment would be evaluated by methods other than testing.

The specification of areas emanate from the objectives which are stated. These objectives must be appropriate to the level of the student and representative of the total array of designated areas of knowledge which can be reasonably expected of the student within that course at the particular time designated for the tests. The process for identifying testable content in an objective is described below. The following is a course objective.

At the conclusion of the course, the student will relate psychosocial concepts to the assessment process of individuals with minimal adaptive needs.

1. AREA TO BE TESTED.

The area to be tested in this objective is:

The relationship between psychosocial concepts and the assessment process.

2. DEFINITION.

The area to be tested within the expected knowledge must be given precise meaning. The precision specifies the types of patient problems to be addressed and the critical elements or test units to be tested. This definition of the area clarifies the limits of inclusion or exclusion and demands that the definition be stated simply and clearly.

Definition of area: psychosocial concepts relevant to the assessment of patients with minimal adaptive needs.

3. CRITICAL ELEMENTS.

The writing of the critical elements or test units derived from the definition of the area calls for behaviors that must be judged in the test. The level behaviors must be specified as acceptable to students at that particular time in their education when the test is administered. These elements or units represent those areas required by all students and the range of acceptability needs to be stated. They must be meaningful, significant, learnable, and centers of concentration and mastery.

It is advisable that a few critical elements or test units for each area be identified so that the emphasis can be addressed to the essentials.

Critical Elements or Test Units

Behavioral: demonstrate relationship
Psychosocial concepts related to minimal adaptive needs:
    antecedent psychological and sociological events
    present psychological and sociological events
    interpersonal actions and meanings
    psychosocial stressors
    psychosocial adaptation

Content then must be addressed to the essentials in nursing practice appropriate to the developmental stage of the student when the test is scheduled. It calls for careful delineation of the critical elements or test units in the area specified by the objectives with those elements expected in the practice of the nurse. The adherence to this last suggestion, behaviors expected by all nursing students, may not be a prerequisite in tests which are designed to discriminate among students in terms of cognitive skills and handling of subject matter. Discriminating tests are norm referenced.

Characteristics

Characteristic concepts of test preparation refer to matters such as sampling, objectivity, acceptability, and comparability. Sampling is concerned with the most frequently encountered areas of nursing care. Questions need to reflect the usual type of nursing action within the framework of the course, not the unusual or esoteric which is out of the province of most students' experience.

In place of objectivity, the term *fair* could be substituted. The careful delineation from the objectives of areas of knowledge and the selection of critical elements or test units should provide questions addressed to essentials that are inherent in the practice of nursing.

Acceptability relates to the expectation of passing if the level is achieved. The baseline is the identification of the critical element or test unit when specified as the basis of nursing practice. Acceptability must be defined in terms of practice and theory, not as the perceived ideal of some faculty member.

Comparability relates to the nature of the test items on tests so that each one calls for the same degree of complexity and demand on the student. In tests where students are provided with choice of test items, this comparability criterion is most important.

Structure and Process

Structure and process relate to the characteristics of consistency, flexibility, and availability of feedback. The concern of consistency relates to consistency among evaluators as well as consistency in the administering of tests. Every effort must be made to assure that there is consistency in interpreting each test. The definition of critical elements or test units with the clearly delineated boundaries of acceptability should be helpful. When there are many evaluators of test items for free response questions, it is advisable that the same person evaluate all student responses on a particular question.

Consistency in the administration of a test is also important, for students need to know the expectations of their behavior during the test situation. Confusion abounds when some faculty in a school proctor tests while other faculty provide no monitoring or supervision. The practice of making available a person to clarify questions during the examination also varies among teachers and creates unnecessary tension and stress for students.

Consistency also relates to the pattern of providing instructions to students relative to their responsibility in responding to questions and their approach to answering the questions. There need not be consistency in test format; as a matter of fact, such a practice would be most destructive to the educational endeavor. However, the student can expect that the instructions will be clearly stated, thereby eliminating the question of whether it is better to guess and answer all questions or to omit questions and answer only those that the student can answer comfortably. The methods of scoring needs to be conveyed to the student on a consistent basis, so that the student can determine the best use of time during the examination process.

Flexibility, the other characteristic of the process, relates to the structure of the test. In a test situation, one can often feel a sense of being confined, with no perceived option to express self or "show what I know." Examinations that provide for choice often give the student some sense of control over the test situation. Choices should not be so numerous that the student spends much time trying to determine what choice to accept. A multiple choice or alternate response question that offers several extra items can often be helpful to a student. An alternate-response format that suggests students choose 10 out of 12 test questions for answering or an essay or problem-solving test which advises the students to select 2 out of 3 or 2 out of 4 questions will provide flexibility which can be supportive of the student.

Flexibility also relates to the interpretation of responses of students. Pre-determined responses are indicated when the test is developed. However, one must approach the interpretation response with a certain degree of humility. Sometimes the student's knowledge base exceeds the teacher's! Opportunity for the student to support a response is important and should be provided in an examination. A well developed or theoretically sound response, although not consistent with the pre-determined criteria, must be accepted. The student who knows he/she has a chance brings a more confident manner to the test situation.

Another factor under process and structure is addressed to the timing for providing feedback of results to students, *availability of results*. The feedback principle is seen within the context of diagnostic teaching. It is advisable that results be available to students within a week of testing. The exact timing is often dependent upon the format of the test and the type of test items to be evaluated. Fixed answer questions, such as multiple choice, alternate response, etc., that can be scored easily may be available for feedback more quickly. Free response questions (essay, problem solving) will necessitate a longer evaluation period, but should still be completed within a week. Final examinations are generally not used for feedback, especially if they are offered during the typical final examination week of a term.

Test Design

An understanding of the process of the development prepares one to consider the actual design of the test. The identification of the objectives to be tested with a clear delineation of the critical elements or test units to be tested requires that the appropriate format for test items be selected.

As mentioned previously, there are two classifications of test items, the fixed answer question and the free response question. The decision as to what format to use depends upon the objectives to be evaluated, the purpose of the examination, the number of students to be tested, and the time required for response analysis. A final examination with the demand for immediate feedback, including a compilation of various evaluation strategies for a course grade to be submitted within forty-eight hours, places real constraints on test makers. With small numbers of students, a free response test may be administered, but with large numbers of students in a limited time frame, the faculty may be forced to rely on fixed answer items.

The expected behavior is critical in selecting the testing format. The behavior signals the point on the taxonomy that the question must address. Generally, fixed response questions are limited to the first three cognitive levels (knowledge, comprehension, and application). Reflective thinking questions are appropriate at most levels beginning with the second one, comprehension. Especially in undergraduate programs the usual test situation does not often go beyond the fourth level, analysis. Affective behaviors may be tested on the first two levels (receiving and responding) by fixed response questions. Free response questions could be used for the second through fourth level (responding, valuing, and organization of values).

One other factor influencing the selection of test items relates to the intent of the examination—criterion referenced or norm referenced. Norm referenced requires that discriminatory items be incorporated. It is generally expected that a discriminatory item be selected so that the top one-third of the students provide a better response than the lower one-third. It must be remembered, however, that the discriminatory question must be derived from the critical element or test unit. Many test makers use this discriminatory process to provide questions outside the expected content area. A discriminatory question needs to address greater depth of one of the critical elements.

The plan of the test is individual in relation to its purpose and the objectives tested. A one-strategy test may be designed or a multi-strategy test may be the appropriate format. The one-strategy test using fixed response questions is easily scorable if it is designed so that the format for response is consistent. It is suggested that the easier items appear first so that the testee feels some sense of achievement on the test. It is difficult to state how many items should be included, generally about 115 items of multiple response are achievable in a two-hour examination period. Again, the number is determined by the level of test items; recall items can be answered more quickly than can those demanding higher cognitive skills.

A single strategy test using free response questions is often more challenging and demanding of the students. The number of test items varies with the objectives to which test items are addressed. A free response question above the first level can often relate to more than one objective.

A multiple-strategy test enables the test designer to test a wider range of behaviors. A variety also relieves the boredom and tendency to answer questions by guessing as the student reaches the final portion of the examination. Boredom facilitates the onset of fatigue during a test situation.

When multiple strategies are used, it is advisable to section the examination, with each section representing a different strategy. Precise instructions for each section must be provided and the weight of each section should be communicated to the student. Choice in questions within each section to be answered is also helpful to a student.

If the multiple-strategies test includes both types of test items, fixed answer and free response, more time must be provided for the free response questions. In a situation test, the items may represent both types of questions—again as determined by the behaviors to be tested. Weighing in multi-strategy tests is most important, with the highest weight assigned to the free response questions unless the latter are only a small part of the test.

Once test items are developed, it might be appropriate to test out the items with faculty, colleagues, or other students not involved in the test situation. This experience often helps to identify any ambiguity in the wording or the conveying of a message not compatible with the original intent for the question. The post-test analysis will be discussed subsequently.

Criteria

In any test development, certain criteria need to be considered in determining its appropriateness for use. Criteria include:

1. Validity — the extent to which the test measures what it is intended to do

2. Reliability — the consistency with which the test measures what it is designed to do

3. Administrability — the ease of administration of the test for both faculty and student

4. Cost Effectiveness — the reasonableness of the cost of the test in relation to its development, administration, analysis, and scoring

5. Scorability — the potential for scoring within the confines of time, faculty ability, and fairness

6. Accuracy in preparation of materials — the preparation of the test with regard to clarity of instruction, accuracy of typing, spacing of items, and facility in recording answers

ETHICAL ISSUES

What value of testing within the educational endeavor was reflected in the behavior of the faculty in the previously described scenario? Do faculty perceive any ethical issues in their behavior?

The significance placed on test performance in society is well recognized. It is acknowledged that because of prevalant testing practices, much unnecessary stress is placed upon the testee as the test situation is encountered. Should an activity so highly significant to the student and surrounded by such social significance be developed so carelessly, without regard to principles of fairness, integrity, and accountability?

No test will be developed that is totally objective. Tests can be developed that are fair in terms of substance and the expectations of the individual to be tested. Does not the student have the *right* to fair testing procedures? Are faculty accountable for assuring that the student's right is being protected? No student should ask "what will be on the test?" Instead the teacher should notify the students about the objectives to be included in a specific test and then develop a test consistent with those objectives.

Will James in 1892 said, "We are all too apt to measure gains for our pupils in their proficiency in directly reproducing in a recitation or on examinations such matters as they may have learned."[4] Is it *reproductive* or *productive* thinking that we are rewarding in our testing endeavors?

SUMMARY

Testing is an integral part of the educational experience, one which can either facilitate or deter the student's learning. Faculty that sincerely answer the three critical questions: Why am I testing? How am I testing? What results am I getting? will design and administer tests that promote the student's desire "to know what I know" rather than a desire to survive the system. Test development is directed by specific purposes and addressed to the essentials. Norm-referenced examinations use a stated norm as a referent while criterion-referenced examinations use an absolute standard as a referent. The latter purpose is most compatible with teacher-developed tests used in a nursing program which stresses competency as the achievement level. All tests must meet criteria of validity, reliability, administrability, cost effectiveness, scorability, and accuracy in preparation of materials.

Because of the significance of testing in our society and the uses of tests in determining directions in life open to individuals, the faculty must be held ethically responsible to protect the rights of the testee. Data obtained by results are significant for inclusion in both formative and summative processes in a course. Tests can be purposeful, creative, challenging, interesting, and informative.

REFERENCES

1. Eble, K. The Craft of Teaching. San Francisco:Jossey-Bass, 1976, p. 102.
2. Brunner, J.S. Process of Education. New York:Vintage Books, 1963, p.52.
3. Lenberg, C. Unpublished Paper Presented at Conference. Albany, N.Y. July 1978.
4. James, W. Talks to Teachers. New York:W.W. Norton, 1959, pp. 100–101.

RECOMMENDED READINGS

Adkins, D.C. Test Construction: Development and Interpretation of Achievement Tests. (5th ed.) Columbus, Ohio:Charles Merrill Co., 1974.

Ainsworth, D. Examining the Basis for Competency Based Education. J. High. Educ. Vol. 48, 3:321, May/June 1977.

Barr, D. Multiple Choice Tests. Columbia U. Forum, VI. 3:32, Summer 1963.

Bloom, B., Hastings, J.T. & Madaus, G.F. Handbook on Formative and Summative Evaluation of Student Learning. New York:McGraw-Hill Co. 1971.

Bloom, B., Krathwohl, D. & Masia, B. Taxonomy of Educational Objectives Handbook I. Cognitive Domain. New York:David McKay Co. 1956.

Bower, F.L. Normative or Criterion Referenced Evaluation? Nurs. Outl., 22:499, 1974.

Friedenberg, E. The Real Functions of Educational Testing. Change, 2:43, January/February 1971.

Kegan, D. Using Bloom's Cognitive Taxonomy for Curriculum Planning and Evaluation in Non-traditional Educational Settings. J. High. Ed., Vol. 48, 2: 63, January/February 1973.

Krumme, A.S. The Case for Criterion-Referenced Measurement, Nurs. Outl., 23:764, 1975.

Lyman, H.B. Test Scores and What They Mean. (2nd ed.) Englewood Cliffs, N.J. Prentice-Hall, Inc., 1971.

Meskauskas, J.A. Evaluation Models for Criterion-Referenced Testing: Views Regarding Mastery and Standard Setting. Rev. Ed. Res., 46: 133, 1976.

Millan, J. Criterion-Referenced Measurement. In Pophan, W.J. (ed): Evaluation in Education: Current Applications, Berkeley, Ca.: McCutchan, 1974, pp. 309-398.

Pophan, W.J. (ed). Criterion-Referenced Measurement. Englewood Cliffs, N.J.: Educational Technology, 1971.

Quiring, J.D. The Level of Questions Posed by Nursing Educators. J. Nurs. Ed. Vol. 12, 3: 15, August 1973.

Reilly, D. (ed.) Teaching and Evaluating the Affective Domain in Nursing Programs. Thorofare, N.J.:Charles B. Slack, 1978.

Rezler, A.G. & Liu, R.W. Hope for the Hopeless Essay Test. J. Nurs. Ed., 16:5, November 1977.

Ross, G.R., Ross, M.C. Using the Computer to Prepare Multiple Choice Examinations: A Simplified System. J. Nurs. Ed., 16:32, May 1977.

Tom, A.R. Critique of Performance Based Teaching Education. Ed. For., 42, 11:77, November 1977.

10 Methods of Evaluating Attainment of Clinical Behavioral Objectives

Teachers in a professional program such as nursing must concern themselves not only with evaluating the student's mastery of behavioral objectives as demonstrated by the usual academic procedures but also must assess the student's competency in actual practice. Professionals practice their discipline and are held accountable for the quality of their practice. Thus the development of practice competency is a critical dimension of any professional program and must be a matter of continuous evaluation.

MEANING OF CLINICAL PRACTICE

Although the term *clinical practice* is familiar to individuals involved in nursing, perceptions of the term vary considerably. To some, it implies a series or an aggregate of tasks; to others, the term implies a process.

Clinical practice may be viewed as the way or the medium through which a professional practitioner ministers to the client. The term *client* is used here instead of *patient* to emphasize nursing's involvement in health maintenance and disease prevention as well as in treatment of illness. Practice methodology represents a specific constellation of practitioner abilities developed through some educational experiences. Thus, clinical practice may be conceptualized as the way the nurse utilizes a particular constellation of abilities to meet the health needs of the client.

Who are the clients? For nursing purposes, clients are individuals, groups, families, or communities. They are any of these representing all ages; any ethnic, religious, or socioeconomic group; as well as degrees of health and various stages of illness. They are any of these in a variety of settings: home, community, health care facilities, schools, businesses, or industry. The nurse meets the client whenever and wherever a health need (health maintenance or illness) exists, and it is to the person with specific health/illness problems that the nurse practitioner addresses his/her practice.

The nature of the relationship of nurse to client and to the problem at hand is an important consideration in defining the term *clinical practice*. Three possible views of this relationship are:

1. The nurse is in a subsidiary role, programmed as a functional agent to do things for the patient and the patient's environment. The nurse in this task-centered relationship uses prescriptions for intervention, designed for particular needs.
2. The nurse relates methods of care to the needs and problems of the client in a particular state of health. The nurse, using a nursing-process approach, views the totality of the client's being and relates professional intervention to the particular needs or problems evident in the client situation.
3. The nurse is a diagnostician, an integral part of the health service situation in which he/she intervenes. The nurse (also process-oriented) is a problem solver who develops a nursing diagnosis, proposes a nursing prescription relative to the diagnosis, and carries out the prescription through to evaluation. In this relationship the nurse is involved in patient-management decisions.

Nurse teachers must develop a concept of clinical practice in terms of the nature of actions involved, the client served, and the relationship of the nurse to the clients and their problems. The concept the teacher holds determines the expectations, the evaluation strategies, and the reward systems associated with clinical practice.

NURSING PROCESS

Nursing process is generally accepted today as the *methodology of nursing*. A process is perceived as a series of actions or operations that are goal directed, sequential, interrelated, and dynamic. Nursing process is a sequential series of planned actions by which the nurse meets the health needs of a client. The process involves:

1. Intellectual operations, such as problem solving, decision making, and application of a synthesis of theories, ideas, and concepts.
2. Value judgments based on the respect of the dignity and worth of man.
3. Psychomotor skills, both for assessment and for intervention.

Since the nursing process is the methodology of practice, the major focal point in evaluating clinical practice is the learner's competency in using the process. Identification of nursing actions implicit in the process serves as the basis for evaluation. The nursing actions are behavioral objectives.

Nursing literature contains many fine references about the nursing process and its implication for nursing practice. The discussion here is aimed at suggesting nursing behaviors inherent in the process that are amenable to evaluation. The classification of steps in the process varies according to the viewpoint of the particular author, but in general the following four steps are identified:

1. Assessment
2. Planning
3. Implementation
4. Evaluation

The following behaviors are suggested for each of the steps in the process.

Assessment

1. Makes relevant observations.
2. Conducts purposeful interviews.
3. Uses appropriate resources for data gathering.
4. Uses technical data gathering skills.
5. Collects data regarding care plans of other health team members.
6. Interprets data in terms of scientific theories, concepts, and principles.
7. Relates client's response to health or illness to the sociocultural background.
8. Accepts the right of clients to their own philosophy, moral code, and life style.
9. Seeks to avoid interference of own biases when interpreting data.
10. Uses appropriate resources for clarification.
11. Identifies client's resources that can be used in meeting health needs.
12. Differentiates between own data analysis and that identified for a "typical situation."
13. Identifies significant relationships from data.
14. Draws conclusions from data relationships.

15. Identifies overt and covert needs.
16. Relates identified needs to care plans of other health-team members.
17. Establishes a priority of needs.
18. Establishes a nursing diagnosis (es) from data.

Planning

1. Involves the client in determining long-and short-term goals.
2. Develops objectives for nursing care based on nursing diagnosis.
3. Involves the client in the development of the plan of care.
4. Relates the nursing care plan to the plan of care by other health team members.
5. Selects nursing measures calculated to be most effective in meeting objectives.
6. Establishes a nursing care plan consistent with objectives.
7. Communicates plan of care to other nursing personnel.

Implementation

1. Carries out nursing measures consistent with scientific concepts.
2. Uses technical skills competently.
3. Maintains a therapeutic environment.
4. Informs client of actions inherent in the therapeutic plan.
5. Uses self therapeutically.
6. Uses appropriate channels for communicating relevant information.
7. Records significant information accurately.
8. Protects the client's right to privacy.
9. Protects legal rights of clients.
10. Encourages clients to utilize own capacities to maximum potential.
11. Assists the client and family to accept realistic limitations imposed by illness.
12. Accepts responsibility to act on behalf of the client when conflict exists between the nurse's and the client's moral and ethical code.
13. Applies appropriate measures to cope with barriers to effective communication.
14. Initiates referrals based on identified needs to selected community resources.
15. Instructs the client and family in relation to identified learning needs.
16. Works with clients and others to provide for continuity of care.

Evaluation

1. Uses criteria to measure the results of nursing intervention in terms of the objectives.

2. Uses evaluative data to assess each step of the process.
3. Modifies plan as indicated in the evaluation.

Inclusion of these behaviors does not suggest that only those behaviors directly associated with the nursing process are to be evaluated in clinical practice. These behaviors are critical if the learner is to demonstrate competence in nursing process, but other behavioral objectives may be of equal import. The behaviors ultimately selected for evaluation in clinical practice arise from behavioral objectives expressed for the program and for that part of the program with which a particular clinical practice is associated.

PURPOSES OF CLINICAL PRACTICE
IN A NURSING PROGRAM

Since nursing is a practice discipline, it requires not only cognitive mastery of relevant theories, but skill in their use within the practice domain. Practice then becomes an essential component of the preparation of the nursing practitioner and must be central to professional education, not peripheral to it.

Many of the implications of the practice component of a professional curriculum have not been carefully analyzed by nursing educators. Argyris and Schön[1] (1974) suggest that the field experience in a professional program should not be designed simply to give students experience in the real world to learn accepted practices, but it should also provide opportunity to try out new modalities of care. Indeed, the real world may reinforce the concept of routinized practice and narrow the student's perspective of the options available to broaden and deepen one's practice.

The use of clinical practice as a means of enabling students to try out new modalities of care requires the acceptance of risk-taking behavior. This behavior is not chance behavior, but a carefully considered plan of action in which possible consequences have been identified, but the actual outcome is uncertain. It is problem-solving behavior. But can faculty support this risk-taking behavior from the students, or do they need the security of known outcome? If faculty do not accept the process of learning as well as the outcome, then they favor imitative practice and do little to encourage the creative potentials of students.

Clinical practice is essential for another purpose in relation to the professional development of potential nursing practitioners. It is a major contribution to the process by which students·learn to *think* like practitioners. It is central to professional education because it facilitates the learning associated with commitment and personal causation, the acceptance of responsibility for what the individual does as a practitioner. Clinical practice, then, is more than the opportunity to put classroom theory into use in the real world; it also provides opportunity for the development of problem-solving and decision-making skills, and the development of attitudes and values reflective of the professional practitioner.

Argyris and Schön caution professional educators about the realistic misfit between the field experience and the structure of institutions of higher learning. Although they acknowledge that practice must play a central role in the process by which students learn to think like practitioners, they remind us that the school cannot claim responsibility for the preparation of all professional competencies. They state, "The variety, duration, and realism of work experience required to provide opportunity for developing the full range of professional competencies are simply incompatible with the boundaries and structure of school experience as it is currently defined. The structure of the school year, the demands on student time made by course work, the boundaries among discipline-oriented departments, the demand of term papers and theses, the ladders of academic security and prestige all limit the intensity and duration of involvement in practice that would enable the student to acquire a full range of professional competence."[2]

Are the authors suggesting that faculty be more realistic in their expectations of practice competence which the graduates are expected to achieve as they leave schools of nursing? Faculty need to explore further this misfit between the demands for acquiring clinical competence and the structural framework within which they seek to assist the learner in developing these competencies.

INFLUENCE OF THE SUPERVISORY PROCESS ON THE EVALUATION OF CLINICAL PRACTICE

Before proceeding to the discussion of strategies appropriate for clinical practice evaluation, it is important to explore the impact of the supervisory process in the clinical field on the evaluation process. The supervisory process, inherent in teaching in the practice field, generates many anxieties that differentiate evaluation of clinical practice from that of the usual academic situation.

Competency in clinical practice demands changes in behavior in all three domains (cognitive, affective, and psychomotor). Moreover, these changes must be demonstrated within the confines of a close relationship with the teacher. The process of change, which often details a period of discomfort as the new approach is being developed, occurs under the watchful eye of an observer, the teacher. Feelings of inadequacy often result, and the learner is vulnerable to fears of criticism, shame, and rejection. The degree to which these fears become operant in the student relates to the student's perception of authority. Indeed, the supervisory relationship may take on the semblance of a parent-child relationship and evoke behavioral responses commensurate with the participants' own experiences. Not only must the learner's process of becoming a practitioner occur within view of the teacher, but it usually occurs within view of many others, such as patients, families, peers, and other professionals.

In clinical evaluation, therefore, the student is even more vulnerable than in the usual educational evaluation situations. Acceptance of the realities of this vulnerability is crucial if evaluation is to be a facilitative process in the student's growth as a practitioner. A supportive climate based on trust and acceptance does much to minimize the negative effects that may result from the anxieties inherent in the evaluation of clinical practice.

If the environment is not supportive, participants in the evaluation process resort to game playing. Kadushin (1968), in his article *Games People Play in Supervision,* describes many of the games that engage the energies of participants. Game playing is adopted because of the payoff. Kadushin has stated, "One party to the game chooses a strategy to maximize his payoff and minimize his penalties. He wants to win rather than to lose, and he wants to win as much as he can at the lowest cost."[3]

If the learners feel threatened they will resort to gamesmanship in an attempt to win the evaluation game. The focus of evaluation becomes survival rather than attainment of behavioral objectives relevant to clinical practice. In other words, evaluation assesses survival, not learning.

METHODS OF EVALUATING CLINICAL PRACTICE

When the expression *clinical practice* is used in nursing, there is a direct association with a piece of paper called an Evaluation Form. The question usually raised is: What one form is best for clinical evaluation? It is interesting that one does not hear the question: What one form is appropriate for class evaluation?

Clinical practice is complex and of course cannot be evaluated by any single procedure. No form by itself is an appropriate evaluative device. The nature of the practice to be assessed is determined by the level of practice expected by the particular type of practitioner involved. If professional practice is the goal, evaluative procedures must discriminate between theoretically based practice and that which is intuitive or imitative. Since the cognitive, affective, and psychomotor domains are encompassed in practice, strategies must be used to insure mastery in all domains.

As with any evaluation, the procedure used is that which provides data relative to the student's progress toward, or attainment of, specified behavioral objectives. Both summative and formative evaluation strategies are in order. However, since clinical practice competency is a developmental process, it is particularly important that a systematic approach to formative evaluation be incorporated into the program.

The focus of clinical practice evaluation is the *student*—and that student's growth toward mastery of practice; thus any evaluation procedure that supplies data for making judgments about the student's practice is appropriate. Many evaluation strategies discussed in the previous chapter are suitable, especially those related to problem-solving, with or without the added dimensions supplied by various forms of multimedia. Pencil and paper tests and written assignments also are useful in determining the cognitive base of student practice and the beliefs and values guiding student responses to the demands of practice. Evaluation procedures particularly identified with clinical practice may be viewed in the following three major classifications:

1. Observation.
2. Written communication.
3. Oral communication.

OBSERVATION METHODS

One of the evaluative procedures of the practice dimension of student learning used most often is the observation of student behavior during nursing actions. The usual means of recording these observations are:

1. Anecdotal notes.
2. Critical incident.
3. Rating scales.

Anecdotal Notes

Anecdotal notes are frequently used in nursing education for recording data about the student's practice, although many nurse teachers have reservations about their validity and reliability. The concerns expressed relate to the format of the note, the system of collecting the notes, and the use made of the information collected.

Perhaps some teachers expect too much from anecdotal notes simply because they do not fully understand their function. An anecdotal note is a recorded description of the behavior and activities of the learner during a particular performance of short duration. It is a vignette of the learner's practice experience. The note itself is usually written informally without modifying expressions and contains only data that clarify the image of the event.

Some individuals enlarge the scope of the anecdotal note by including an interpretation of it, or by making inferences from the event. This approach detracts from the principal function of anecdotal notes. If interpretation is desired, it should be included in a notation separate from the description and provision should be made for the learner to include a personal interpretation.

The system to be used in collecting anecdotes causes much concern among nurse teachers, primarily because most attempts result in an erratic pattern. Generally speaking, faculty end up with many notes for some students (especially students having difficulty) and few notes for others, with inequities among students in the behaviors selected for recording and inconsistencies in the numbers of notes collected during various periods in the practice term. Indeed, the quantity and quality of notes may reflect the mood and interest of the evaluator. They also neglect the influence of factors such as time and other demands being made upon the evaluator.

Many of these problems can be eliminated if a systematic approach is developed for the collection of anecdotal notes. When behavioral objectives are identified for clinical practice, nurse teachers should make decisions as to how each is to be evaluated. At that time, certain behaviors can be selected for evaluation by anecdotal notes, and the number of notes to be selected for each student can be stated. Thus, all students will be evaluated on the same behavioral objectives by the same number of notes. This system also helps the faculty to be realistic about the number of notes it is possible to collect in any clinical practice period. This decision by no means limits the number of notes a teacher may write. The teacher can still use personal judgment about the need to obtain more data about some students. The student, however, should be informed about the increase in the number of anecdotal notes to be written and should know the rationale underlying the decision.

ILLUSTRATIONS

BEHAVIORAL OBJECTIVE	EVALUATION
A3.2 Assumes responsibility for explaining procedures to a school age child before beginning the task.	In 2 out of 3 observations recorded in anecdotal notes, the student explains the procedure. *Criteria for evaluation* 1. Explanation precedes the start of the procedure 2. Explanation is in language understandable to the child 3. Explanation is accurate 4. Child is encouraged to ask questions and express concerns 5. Questions are answered accurately and sensitively
P4.0 Uses auscultation technique accurately.	In 3 out of 4 observations recorded on anecdotal notes, the student uses auscultation technique accurately.

BEHAVIORAL OBJECTIVE   EVALUATION

Criteria for evaluation
1. Identifies the proper landmark
2. Uses stethoscope properly
3. Distinguishes sounds correctly
4. Carries out procedure within a reasonable time frame

These two illustrations demonstrate a use for anecdotal notes. The anecdotes are recorded and the teacher and learner evaluate recorded behaviors according to stated criteria. This process is most effective in formative evaluation, but the quantification criterion makes it possible to use anecdotal notes in a summative evaluation.

Anecdotal notes are valuable in recording longitudinal data about the student's progress in developing practice competency. However, there must be a systematic plan so that there are no gaps in recording, for a sufficient number of notes must be collected at regular intervals to describe the developmental process accurately. The quantitative demands of this approach, especially if large numbers of students are involved, often impede the data gathering necessary for the qualitative judgments required for a longitudinal study.

Critical Incident Technique

This technique was discussed in the previous chapter as a method of assessing the student's analytic and problem-solving competencies. In the practice area, the critical incident involving some aspect of the student's performance can be recorded and performance evaluated according to stated criteria.

The concept of a critical incident differs from that of an anecdote. Fivars and Gosnell (1966) define a critical incident as "one that makes a significant difference in the outcome of an activity. It may be the positive factors that contribute towards the success of the behavior or it may be the negative factors that interfere with the completion of the assignment."[4] Anecdotes, on the other hand, are not selected because they have implications for outcome, but because they are relevant to the behavioral objective being evaluated. The reader is referred to *Nursing Evaluation: The Problem and the Process* for more detailed information on the critical incident technique.

Use of the critical incident technique as a data gathering mechanism could be similar to that for the anecdotal record. Specific behavioral objectives would be identified as particularly amenable to evaluation by critical incident. The criteria for analysis of incidents, however, would be stated also in terms of student behaviors influencing outcomes of the activity positively or negatively.

Illustration

BEHAVIORAL OBJECTIVE	EVALUATION
C3.0 Shares own assessment of patient needs with colleagues in the nursing team.	Two critical incident reports from team conferences.

Criteria for evaluation
1. Identify
    a. learner behaviors which assisted team members in understanding patient needs
    b. learner behaviors which interfered with the team members' understanding of patient needs

The critical incident technique is effective for formative evaluation; it enables the learner and the teacher to assess the learner's behaviors in relation to their impact on the outcome of an action. It can also be used in summative evaluation, provided several critical incidents are used to judge the student's mastery of the behavior under consideration.

Rating Scales

Rating scales continue to be a part of the evaluation process for nursing practice in many situations. Unfortunately, rating scales have been misused and have often been *the* method used to evaluate practice, to the exclusion of other strategies. When the request for a form for practice evaluation is made, it is often a search for a rating scale. The impossible search continues for the one perfect rating scale, which infallibly will convey the degree of competency the practitioner has achieved.

It is important to know what is meant by a rating scale. Technically, it is a standardized device for recording qualitative and quantitative judgments about *observed* performance. It contains a list of traits, activities, skills, or attitudes that may or may not be stated behaviorally. The evaluator is asked to rate, according to best judgment, the learner's competency for each item on some point on a continuum, such as excellent-poor, achieved-not-achieved, etc. In general, rating scales with behaviorally expressed items are more helpful than those with items expressed as a list of traits; the behaviors are less ambiguous.

Rating scales have certain limitations that must be considered when a practice evaluator is determining their use within a program. Since the scales are standardized procedures, the items (behaviors) listed may or may not be consistent with stated objectives for a particular course or learning experience. The teacher must analyze the behaviors in relation to their relevancy to objectives being evaluated, so that the rating scale selected will include statements of behaviors that at least approximate expected outcomes of the learning experience. Some behaviors on the scale may be discounted if they are not relevant.

Another limitation is the lack of uniformity with which terms are interpreted by evaluators. This is particularly true with terms used to designate various intervals in the rating continuum. An operational definition that includes illustrations of acceptable behaviors for each interval can facilitate reliability.

One of the major limitations reflects the interests and values of evaluators. Since some form of "checking off" is called for, some evaluators tend to place checks in some intervals without really doing the essential appraisal. The checking may represent a halo effect whereby the evaluator selects an interval on the continuum on the basis of prior knowledge, personal biases, or close identification with the learner. Scales that call for supportive statements to justify the interval selection help to decrease this halo effect.

The items themselves may limit the use of rating scales since they usually represent the multidimensional character of practice and all items may not be of equal importance. Thus, the value inconsistency among the items in the composite make it inadvisable to use the scale quantitatively.

Rating scales do have a very important place in the schema for practice evaluation. They represent descriptive data of performance that suggest areas of strengths and weaknesses. They may be employed to rate an observed performance or they may be used as a summary description of performance. If used to rate an observed performance, it is important that each learner be rated more than once, for the pattern, rather than one single episode, of behavior is significant. Used in this manner, a record is made of what the learner does; the scale does not discriminate among theoretically based, imitative, and intuitive behaviors.

Rating scales, however, can be most effective in presenting data about all aspects of student practice at periodic intervals. Faculty could even devise their own rating scale from behaviors they have specified for a program, course, or unit of study. Used in this fashion, the rating scale could exhibit a profile of student performance during regularly scheduled time periods. Such a profile would be a useful tool in helping the learner as well as the teacher identify areas of practice to be supported or to be strengthened. Used with different color markings for each evaluation period this scale helps to present a picture of the student's developmental process. In this use of the scale, teachers must define the data base they will use and strategies for obtaining the data, so that markings on the scale will reflect the student's total learning experience.

Rating scales are evaluative devices that are addressed to a composite of rather than to one specific behavior. They are most effective in the system for formative evaluation. Due to irregularities in the value of different items, rating scales ordinarily are not properly subject to the grading process.

WRITTEN COMMUNICATION METHODS

Nurses communicate among themselves and among practitioners of other disciplines through the written media; various forms of written communication serve as significant evaluation strategies. In this type of evaluation, one is concerned with two dimensions: skill in communicating and quality of the substance communicated. The usual methods are:

1. Nurses' notes
2. Problem oriented records
3. Nursing care studies
4. Process recording

Nurses' Notes

The ability to report and record nursing actions is identified as a critical behavior in most nursing programs, yet the medium for most of this reporting and recording, the patient's chart, has seldom been used in a systematic evaluation protocol of learner practice competency. The learner has been expected to write in the nurses' notes, but evaluative data about the student's clinical practice performance seldom reflect skill in recording and the quality of the substance recorded.

The significance of the patient's chart is becoming increasingly apparent as the movement to demand accountability for quality health care gains momentum. Phaneuf (1972) has devised a nursing audit protocol for ascertaining quality nursing care based on the use of the patient's chart as the source of data. Her rationale for using the patient's chart as the source of information is: "The chart is a service instrument essential to the safety of the patient and the management of care. It serves as the major means of communication between the various professionals involved in the care. It provides legal documentation of care provided. Recording is a part of one of the seven functions of nursing. The chart is readily available to authorized nurses for purposes of auditing."[5]

Use of the patient's chart in quality control and the present impetus toward problem-oriented records demand that greater emphasis in clinical practice be placed on the recording competencies of the nurse. If the recording is to be seen as an integral part of the total care of the patient, and not some routine activity to be accomplished before one leaves the practice unit, then the learner's recording behaviors must be carefully assessed.

Nursing care, which is process-oriented, requires considerable intradisciplinary and interdisciplinary communication so that the integrity and continuity of patient care can be maintained. Therefore, the student's communication behavior must be evaluated systematically. Criteria for evaluating the recording competency refer to the substance of the record and the skill in the technique. Substance deals with facts included and quality of implications derived from the facts. Phaneuf defines essential facts as "those indispensable to patient-centered care, as well as those that are clinically significant as discrete facts."[6] Critical to the substance is the nurse's judgment relative to the meaning of facts in terms of patient needs and essential care. Therefore criteria relate to the appropriateness and comprehensiveness of significant facts, the accuracy of data collection and interpretation, and the consistency with which reported plans and actions are congruent with assessment data.

Skill in communication concerns the degree to which the nurse conveys the message to the reader. This skill encompasses clarity of terminology and composition, conciseness of the message, and logic in ordering elements of the message.

The data gathered for this recording competency may include several longitudinal studies in which the student's recordings of a patient are analyzed over a period of time, or it may represent a certain number of recordings of patients at a particular interval in the learning experience. The design used depends upon the objective of the experience.

Problem-Oriented Records

Recognition of the importance to patient care of an orderly system of written communication among professionals, in the light of the increase in numbers of practitioners involved with any one patient's care, has given impetus to the movement toward problem-oriented records.

A problem-oriented record is perceived as a systematic record keeping centered around the patient's health problems. As delineated by Weed[7] (1969), it consists of the four following major components:

1. Data base: all appropriate information about patient for assessing his condition.
2. Problem list: listing the conditions, systems, or circumstances identified from the data base, which have implications for the patient's health. Each problem is numbered.
3. Initial plans: diagnostic and therapeutic orders for each problem listed. Plans are keyed to each problem.
4. Progress notes:
   a. Narrative note—an expository comment relative to each problem.
   b. Flow sheets—graphic forms to record repetitive and serial data.
   c. Discharge summary—follow-up organized around each problem.

This approach to record keeping is integrative, as all professionals involved in the patient's care participate in developing and maintaining the record. Recording is also integrative rather than segregative, as in the usual form of patient charts which contain nurses' notes, doctors' notes, laboratory reports, etc. The focus is the patient and his/her problems; each individual is regarded as a totality.

The system designed for the problem-oriented record reports more than the events relative to the patient. It also conveys the rationale of practitioners so that there is a better understanding of therapeutic actions. Such exposure, however, leaves individuals vulnerable to challenge by other team members. This challenge holds the individual accountable for decisions and actions and further helps to eliminate routinized or stereotypic types of recordings so frequently found in patient records.

Since the report of actions and the thoughts behind the actions are a vital part of the record, problem-oriented records are a valuable learning experience of the nursing learner. They are compatible with the nursing process as the methodology of nursing. They become an important evaluation device for determining the student's competency in collecting data, identifying problems from the data, and developing relevant plans for care as well as the skill in recording patient progress in terms of specified problems. An additional dimension to student evaluation is possible with problem-oriented records. Since all relevant health-team members also record in the same record, it is possible to assess the learner's ability to relate individual plans and actions to those of other participants in the patient's care.

As with any written communication, not only the quality of the substance the student includes in the record, but also skill in communicating the message must be considered in assessing the student's competency with problem-oriented recording. This evaluation strategy has much value in formative evaluation, especially when accompanied by individual conferences.

Nursing Care Studies

The nursing care study is a familiar evaluation strategy in nursing education programs, although the form and intent may vary considerably. Schweer (1972) defines a nursing care study as "a problem-solving activity whereby the student undertakes the comprehensive assessment of a particular patient's problems leading to planning, implementing, and evaluating of nursing care measures."[8] It is an individualized approach to learning and is often used for independent study in the clinical area.

The traditional form of nursing care study presents a holistic concept of nursing care and is particularly valuable in evaluating the student's competency in the nursing process. The student's written description of actions implicit in meeting patient needs enables the evaluator to determine ability not only in cognitive and affective domains for each step of the process but the ability to establish meaningful relationships among steps of the process. The complexity of the problem situation in terms of nursing judgments and decisions is determined by the level of behaviors expressed for the experiences. A study designed at a comprehensive level calls for interpretative and extrapolative behaviors—behaviors very different from those required at the analytic cognitive level.

In selecting a care study method for the learner, it must be certain that the nature of the problem to be addressed and the number of variables with which the learner must deal are within the student's educational level. This means that behavioral objectives must be clearly stated and relevant to behavioral objectives of the course or unit of study. Evaluation, as with other forms of written communications, is in terms of substance and skill in the communication technique.

Modifications of the nursing-care study should be encouraged so that the learner does not view the study as an end rather than as a means to an end. Other forms of problem-solving strategies, as discussed in the previous chapter, can be used to modify the care study, providing the problem is derived from the student's practice experience.

Process Recording

A procedure that has an important place in any systematic scheme for formative evaluation is the nursing process recording. The evaluative approach is directed toward the learner's behaviors in interactions with others. Schweer defines the process recording as the "verbatim, serial reproduction of the verbal and nonverbal communications between two individuals for the purpose of assessing interactions on a continuum leading toward mutual understanding and interpersonal relationships."[9]

Process recording is amenable to any interaction of the learner with another individual, such as the learner and client, the learner and a health-team member, and between learner and learner. The most frequent use for the process recording is in nurse-patient interactions.

There are various formats for recording such communications, but in general there are four main components:

1. Client communication.
2. Nurse communication.
3. Nurse's interpretation of patient communication.
4. Implications of the communication for nursing actions.

Nursing Process Recording

Client Communication	Nurse Communication	Nursing Interpretation	Implications for Nursing Actions

Client communication includes a verbatim report of all verbal and non-verbal behaviors of the client. The nurse's communication includes verbatim verbal and nonverbal behaviors of the nurse, inclusive of conscious feelings and actions. Nursing interpretation states what the nurse perceives as the client's feelings and the meanings of verbal and nonverbal actions. Implications for nursing actions are derived from the nurse's judgment of the meaning of the client's as well as his/her own communication.

A process recording is best used in conjunction with the individual conference approach, so that the teacher and the learner can evaluate the total interaction as well as each of its component parts. This procedure is especially suitable for formative evaluation, for it is carried out during the learning process and provides for diagnosis and remedial measures.

The total procedure is a time-consuming one and therefore the quantity per learning experience needs to be kept within reasonable limits. The behavioral objective(s) must be sharply defined so that the student focuses on the interaction. The report should be written immediately after the interaction occurs, while the event is vivid in the learner's memory. The teacher's evaluation and the conference should be held within a short time (at the most one week) after the event, so the learner can use the assessment in the development of interpersonal relations skills.

ILLUSTRATION

BEHAVIORAL OBJECTIVE

A3.3 Encourages the patient to express fears and concerns about impending surgery.

C3.0 Identifies verbal and nonverbal clues of patient.

C3.0 Relates nursing actions to identified patient clues.

EVALUATION PROCEDURE

Process recording of nurse-patient interaction in the preoperative period.

Criteria for evaluation
1. Identification of patient verbal and nonverbal cues
2. Identification of own verbal and nonverbal cues
3. Appropriateness of interpretation of patient behaviors
4. Relevancy of implications for nursing actions to cues exhibited in the communications

Process recording, when used with the individual conference, enables the learner to gain skill in analyzing the interaction in terms of the elements. As this skill is developed to a competency level, the learner becomes adept at recognizing inconsistencies and misunderstandings in a communication. This evaluative process is particularly effective in assisting the learner to identify his/her own patterns of behavior in an interaction and thus to become self-evaluative about individual interpersonal relationship skills.

ORAL COMMUNICATION METHODS

Nurses communicate not only through the written media, but they must also be able to convey their ideas and thinking through the spoken word. This ability is of particular importance when presenting information or sharing in the decision-making process with intraprofessional and interprofessional colleagues. The usual methods are:

1. Nursing patient care conferences.
2. Team conferences.

Nursing Patient Care Conferences

Nursing patient care conferences take various forms, but in general they are problem-solving group discussions about some facet of clinical practice. In one format, the student represents a patient situation to the peer group for critical analysis of the plan of action or its implication. The peers evaluate the actions, raise relevant questions, and propose appropriate alternatives. In some instances the conferences may be preceded by nursing rounds in which participants have the opportunity to observe the patients whose nursing care will be discussed.

Other conferences may be less structured and obtain substance from the learner's activities of the day. In this conference format, problems with which the learners are currently engaged are presented for group participation in proposing solutions.

Regardless of format, when group conferences are used in the evaluation schema, the teacher is concerned not only with the quality of the substance and the skillful use of communication techniques (as with written communication methods), but also with the learner's ability to use the group process. Nursing for the most part involves groups, and it is essential that behaviors relevant to individual participation in group process be identified and evaluated. The conference provides an excellent medium for formative evaluation of the student in his or her development in the skills in group work.

Conferences are primarily problem-solving experiences, and the conferences can accordingly be addressed to a particular behavioral objective or to several objectives.

ILLUSTRATIONS

BEHAVIORAL OBJECTIVES	EVALUATION PROCEDURE

C4.2 Relates the plan of nursing action to the hospitalized patient's adaptive response to stress.

C3.0 Uses leadership principles in assisting the conference members to reach nursing managerial decisions.

Nursing Care Conference
1. Student presentation of the stress-adaptation phenomenon as operant in a hospitalized patient

2. Student leadership of group in arriving at nursing managerial decisions

Criteria for evaluation
1. Clarity and comprehensiveness of the identification of stressors
2. Accuracy and completeness of the explanation of demands placed on the patient by these stressors
3. Clarity and comprehensiveness of the identification of patient adaptive behavior
4. Leadership in involving group members in managerial decisions
5. Relevance of decisions to the patient's adaptive response

The nursing care conference is a valuable evaluation strategy and may be used as either a formative or a summative evaluation procedure.

Nursing Team Conference

The team conference is another small group activity that serves as an effective medium for evaluating clinical practice. The composition of the team may vary, ranging from a nursing team made up of practitioners in a particular clinical setting to a highly organized multidisciplinary team in a health-care agency or in a community. The definition of membership is also variable. In some situations, a health team is composed of health-care professionals only; in other situations patients and/or community representatives are included as health-team members.

Whatever the composition of the team, the process in which it is engaged is essentially the same, i.e., shared managerial decision making. Managerial decisions as defined by Feinstein (1970) are "decisions for therapeutic interventions, or to prevent or alter disease."[10] The learner's participation may range from a sharing process to the highly developed skill of collaboration.

The nature of the participation is determined by the stated behavioral objective for the experience.

The most common team activity is problem solving in which, through group process, plans for patient care are developed according to stated patient goals. Implementation of the plan is examined and evaluated for its effectiveness. The learner is evaluated in terms of participation in the group in reporting observations, making relationships among data, making proposals for action, and evaluating actions as they are reported.

ILLUSTRATION

BEHAVIORAL OBJECTIVE	EVALUATION PROCEDURE
C4.3 Collaborates with nursing team members in managerial decisions for a patient.	Team Conference Presentation to nursing team of a patient situation necessitating decisions for a plan for management.

Criteria for evaluation
1. Collects data from other team members
2. Reports own observations
3. Shares with group in interpreting data
4. Shares with group in establishing relationships among data
5. Provides for all members to contribute ideas relative to goals for care
6. Leads group to consensus of goals
7. Listens to members' suggestions for implementation strategies
8. Develops plan of care for patient relevant to needs on the basis of group consensus

Evaluative data about the student in the situation described above may be obtained through the evaluator's observation of the student's behavior, through evaluation reports submitted by team members, through study of a tape recording, or through a videotape of theconference. The results of the evaluation may be used in formative or summative evaluation.

MULTIPLE APPROACHES TO CLINICAL EVALUATION

This chapter has dealt with some of the possible strategies that may be used in evaluating the learner's practice. Actually the extent of the range of strategies is limited only by the teacher's creativity and willingness to take risks and become innovative.

One of the greatest dangers in clinical evaluation is the tendency of the teacher to "get into a rut" with evaluation procedures and to use the same process in each evaluation period with every student. As the approach becomes routinized, practice evaluation becomes an end in itself, divorced from the excitement of learning.

Behavioral objectives, as described and used in this book, are open-ended to encourage teachers to develop their own evaluation strategies. The following example illustrates several approaches that may be used to evaluate a particular behavioral objective.

ILLUSTRATION

BEHAVIORAL OBJECTIVE

C3.0   Conducts purposeful interviews.

EVALUATION METHODS

Possible Approaches
1. Observation by the evaluator
2. Tape recording
3. Videotaping
4. Written interview report
5. Clinical conference

Criteria for evaluation
1. Clear definition of purpose
2. Questions related to purpose
3. Questions stated to elicit responses relevant to purpose
4. Questions comprehensive in scope
5. Responses of patient consistent with scope
6. Patient cues acknowledged
7. Nurse's evaluation of interview in terms of principles of interviewing

It will be noted that five evaluation strategies for the single behavioral objective are suggested. The teacher can vary the strategies with different groups of students, so that they are not confined to one method and thus run the risk of becoming bored and automatic in the preparation of evaluation reports.

The suggestion of the five methods is especially important, however, in enabling the teacher to individualize evaluation procedures. Different methods may be used with different students, according to their needs and the situation in which they are practicing. Another dimension of this individuality relates to the evaluation strategy for summative evaluation.

Although educators profess a belief in individualized learning, they generally require all students to "march to the same drummer" as far as evaluation is concerned. A teacher who adopts a mastery-of-learning approach does not conclude that a student is incapable of meeting the objective on the basis of performance on one evaluation strategy. In the illustration, if the written report of the interview is selected as the evaluation strategy and a student's report is unacceptable, should one then conclude that the student is incapable of conducting a purposeful interview? A mastery-of-learning teacher would select another evaluation procedure before drawing such a conclusion. Perhaps a tape recording or a videotape of an interview would provide evidence that the student could meet the objective.

The suggestion here is that teachers recognize the complex nature of practice and accordingly diversify their evaluation strategies so that the learner and the teacher engage in a developmental rather than a controlling process.

SUMMARY

Evaluation of the learner's clinical practice is a critical element in professional educational programs. The practice of a professional is a complex process by which he/she ministers to the needs of clients. Nursing process is the methodology of nursing practice and represents a composite of cognitive, affective, and psychomotor behaviors. Clinical practice within a nursing education program serves many purposes which must be recognized by faculty.

Evaluation of the learner's practice skills occurs in an environment with built-in threats and pressures. Not only does the supervisory process, by its nature, generate anxieties, but the process takes place in an environment that makes the learner particularly vulnerable. The developmental process that changes behavior takes place in full view of patients, colleagues, and other health workers. Care must be taken that game playing is not resorted to as a means of lessening threats in the clinical field.

The multiplicity of abilities called upon in effective nursing practice demands diverse clinical evaluation strategies. No one procedure is suitable for assessing the totality of practice. Strategies chosen should reflect the particular behavioral objectives to be evaluated, the needs of the learner, and the character of the practice setting.

Procedures suitable for clinical practice evaluation include:

1. Observation (anecdotal notes, critical incident, rating scales).
2. Written communication (nurses' notes, problem-oriented record, nursing care studies, process recording).
3. Oral communication (nursing patient care conference, team conference).

REFERENCES

1. Argyris, C, Schön,D. A Theory in Practice: Increasing Professional Effectiveness. San Francisco: Jossey-Bass, 1974, p. 188.
2. *Ibid,* p. 186.
3. Kadushin, A. Games People Play in Supervision. Social Work, 13:23, 1968.
4. Fivars, G. Gosnell, D. Nursing Evaluation: The Problem and the Process. New York: Macmillan, 1966, p. 159.
5. Phaneuf, M. The Nursing Audit Profile for Excellence. New York: Appleton-Century-Crofts, 1972, p. 32.
6. Idem. p. 50.
7. Weed, L.L. Medical Records, Medical Education, and Patient Care (2nd ed.). Cleveland: The Press of Case Western Reserve University. Distributed by Year Book Medical Publishers, Inc. 1969, p. 13.
8. Schweer, J.E. Creative Teaching in Clinical Nursing (2nd ed). St. Louis: Mosby, 1972, p. 166.
9. Idem. p. 167.
10. Feinstein, A.R. What Kind of Basic Science for Clinical Medicine? N. Engl. J. Med., 283:847, 1970.

RECOMMENDED READINGS

American Nurses Association: Standards, Nursing Practice. Kansas City, Mo.American Nurses Association, 1973.

Berne, E. Games People Play. New York:Grove Press, 1964.

Bloch, D. Evaluation of Nursing Care in Terms of Process and Outcomes. Nurs. Res., 24(4) 256, July/August 1975.

Bower, F.L. The Process of Planning Nursing Care: A Theoretical Model. St. Louis:Mosby, 1972.

Breton, P. The Assessment and Development of Professionals: Theory and Practice. Seattle, Wash.University of Washington, 1976.

Dwyer, J. & Schmitt, J. Using the Computer to Evaluate Clinical Performance. Nurs. For., 8:266, 1969.

Evaluation of Nursing Education Achievement. Report of CENTO Workshop, Ankara, Turkey, 1973.

Hayter, J. An Approach to Laboratory Evaluation. J. Nurs. Educ., 12:17, November 1973.

Hilger, E.E. Developing Nursing Outcome Criteria. Nurs. Clin. N. Amer., 9:323–330, 1974.

Huckabay, L. Cognitive and Affective Consequences of Formative Evaluation in Graduate Nursing Students. Nurs. Res., Vol. 27, 3:190, May/June 1978.

Hurst, J.W. & Walker, H.K. The Problem Oriented System. New York:Med-Com, 1972.

Infante, M.S. The Clinical Laboratory in Nursing Education. New York:Wiley, 1975.

Lenburg, Carrie B. The Clinical Performance Examination. New York: Appleton-Century-Crofts, 1979.

Levine, S. Performance Evaluation. Sup. Nurse, 26-28, 32, 35, 41. September 1977.

Little, D. & Carnevali, D. Nursing Care Planning. Philadelphia:Lippincott 1976.

Longo, D.C. & Williams R.A. Clinical Practice in Psychosocial Nursing: Assessment and Intervention. New York:Appleton-Century-Crofts, 1978.

Maas, M. & Jacox, A. Guidelines for Nurse Autonomy/Patient Welfare. New York:Appleton-Century-Crofts, 1977.

Mager, R.F. & Pipe, P. Analysing Performance Problems. Belmont, California:Lear Siegler/Fearon, 1970.

Mayers, M., Norby, R. & Watson, A. Quality Assurance for Patient Care. New York:Appleton-Century-Crofts, 1977.

Mayers, M.G. A Systematic Approach to the Nursing Care Plan. (2nd ed.) New York:Appleton-Century Crofts, 1978.

Mitchell, P.H. A Systematic Nursing Progress Record: The Problem Oriented Approach. Nurs. For., 12:187, 1973.

Morgan, M.K. & Irby, D.M. Evaluating Clinical Competence in the Health Professions. St. Louis:Mosby, 1978.

Murchison, I., Nichols, T. & Hanson, R. Legal Accountability in the Nursing Process. St. Louis:Mosby, 1978.

Orlando, I.J. The Discipline and Teaching of Nursing Process. New York:G.P. Putnam, 1972.

Phaneuf, M.C. The Nursing Audit: Self-regulation in Nursing Practice (2nd ed). New York:Appleton-Century-Crofts, 1977.

Ryden, M.B. The Predictive Value of a Clinical Evaluation of Interpersonal Relationships Skills. J. Nurs. Ed., Vol 16, 5:77, May 1977.

Schell, P.L., & Campbell, A.T. POMR—Not Just Another Way to Chart. Nurs. Outl. 20:510, 1972.

Schneider, Harriet L. Evaluation of Nursing Competence. Boston:Little, Brown, 1979.

Schweer, J.E. & Gibbie, K.M. Creative Teaching in Clinical Nursing. (2nd ed.) St. Louis:Mosby, 1976.

Schwirian, P.M. Evaluating the Performance of Nurses: A Multidimensional Approach. Nurs. Res. Vol. 27, 6: 347, 1978.

Shostrom, E. Man the Manipulator. New York: Bantam, 1968.

Smith, D. Effect of Values on Clinical Teaching. In J. Williamson (ed): Current Perspectives in Nursing. St. Louis:Mosby, 1976.

Smith, D.W. Perspectives on Clinical Teaching. New York:Springer, 1968.

Wandelt, M.A. & Stewart, D. S. Slater Nursing Competencies Rating Scale. New York:Appleton-Century-Crofts, 1975.

Wandelt, M.A. & Agree, J.W. The Quality Patient Care Scale. New York:Appleton-Century-Crofts, 1974.

Wiedenbach, E. Clinical Nursing; A Helping Art. New York:Springer, 1964.

Wood, V. Casebook in Nursing Education, Ontario: Faculty of Nursing. University of Western Ontario, 1972.

Woody, M. & Mallison, M. The Problem-Oriented System for Patient-Centered Care. Am. J. Nurs., 73:1168, 1973.

Woolley, A. The Long and Tortured History of Clinical Evaluation. Nurs. Outl. Vol. 25, 5:308, May 1977.

Yura, H., Walsh, M. The Nursing Process (3rd ed). New York:Appleton-Century-Crofts, 1978.

Yura, H. & Walsh, M. Human Needs and the Nursing Process. New York:Appleton-Century-Crofts, 1978.

Zimmer, M.J. A Model for Evaluating Nursing Care. Hospitals. 48 (5) 91, 131, March 1974.

11 Behavioral Objectives and Evaluation— Accountability

The concept of instructional accountability was introduced in the beginning of this book. Inherent in this concept is the need for some type of quality control. In instructional endeavors, quality control is addressed to two critical dimensions: relevancy of the instruction and responsibility for the quality of the instruction. As stated in Chapter 1, instructional accountability is one aspect of program accountability. The latter also deals with such matters as the student's own evaluation, the process itself, and the determination of the rightness of objectives. Instructional accountability relates to the question of attainment or nonattainment of the stated goal of the educational experience.

NATURE OF THE RELATIONSHIP BETWEEN THE WHAT AND THE HOW

Any plan designed to ascertain the quality of the instructional effort must be concerned with two variables: the WHAT (behavioral objectives) and the HOW (evaluation strategies). These two variables, however, must not be viewed as separate entities, for it is the relationship between the two variables that influences the reliability and validity of the accountability process. Precisely stated, relevant behaviors have little import if the strategies for evaluating their attainment are not appropriate. Further, well constructed and creative evaluation procedures are meaningless if not directed toward specific behavioral objectives designed for a particular learning endeavor.

The relationship between the WHAT and the HOW is an interdependent one. When behavioral objectives for a learning experience are stated, the underlying assumption is that they will be attained by most learners. Proper testing for achievement depends on the use of appropriate evaluation processes. Evaluation strategies gain their significance from stated behavioral objectives.

Nevertheless this relationship is not an automatic, highly structured one in which a known behavioral objective is associated with a known evaluative strategy. It cannot be diagrammed as Behavioral Objective → Evaluation Strategy, similar to the familiar Stimulus → Response diagram. Operating within this relationship are teachers and learners and all their potentials for creativity. The relationship is a dynamic one, responsive to novelty, change, and environmental stressors.

The relationship is in reality a creative one in which the teacher and the learner are free to explore their own ideas and to interject new approaches. As long as the integrity of the relationship is maintained, the methodology for demonstrating the relationship is open to examination and to trial.

The relationship should be an exciting one for teacher and learner. Variety and novelty can be stimuli for involvement so that assessment of learning does not become an end in itself but an integral part of the instructional process and an opportunity for self-knowledge. When the intent of the relationship between the *what* and the *how* is clear to all participants in the instructional endeavor, the freedom to develop the relationship in a meaningful way presents a challenge. Although the teacher must ultimately be held accountable for the relevance and quality of the instruction, student participation in developing the relationship between behavioral objectives and the strategies for their assessment helps the learner to recognize those aspects of the learning process for which one must be held accountable. Therefore accountability becomes a shared responsibility, demanding specific commitment from all participants.

RELATIONSHIP OF THE CLINICAL AND THE CLASS EVALUATION OF A BEHAVIORAL OBJECTIVE

Professional education must provide evaluation schema not only for the academic situation usually associated with higher education, but also for situations in which the learner can demonstrate ability in those competencies associated with the practice of a chosen profession. The two schema, however, do not imply that two separate sets of behavioral objectives are necessarily indicated. Since professional education is comprised of all three domains of learning (cognitive, affective, and psychomotor), many behavioral objectives may be evaluated in both the classroom and the practice settings.

Behavioral objectives that are open-ended provide clues to evaluation strategies but do not prescribe them. Thus the teacher and, in some cases, the learner are free to develop alternative approaches, providing they maintain the relationship of the evaluation procedure to the stated behavior.

Illustration

BEHAVIORAL OBJECTIVE	CLASS EVALUATION	CLINICAL EVALUATION
C2.2 Describes the influence of emotions on communication.	Listen to four tapes of the interaction of two individuals. Each tape represents a dialogue characterized by one of the following emotions: love, anger, distrust, fear.	Make *two* observations of communication between a patient and a staff member or between two patients in which one of the following four emotions is present: love, anger, distrust, fear.
	Select two of the communication episodes and describe in writing the effect of the emotion on: Voice tone Content Flow of communication Ending of communication	Describe in writing the effect of emotion on: Voice tone Content Flow of communication Ending of communication

In this illustration, data relative to the student's mastery of the behavioral objective may be secured from the class setting and from the clinical setting. One evaluative approach is suggested here for each, but most readers could think of many other strategies for testing this behavior in each area. The class evaluation might be conducted in class or it might be an out-of-class assignment. The clinical evaluation is suggested as a written communication, but it could also be an oral communication in which the student could present the findings at a nursing conference. Not only could the method vary, but the task could vary. There are innumerable ways to assess this behavior and it is up to the teacher to devise different approaches. Diversity is the challenge of evaluation.

Additional Illustrations

BEHAVIORAL OBJECTIVE	CLASS EVALUATION	CLINICAL EVALUATION
C4.1 Identifies feelings of an individual who has venereal disease.	*Essay Question* Cindy Smith, age 16, has just been told by a physician that she has gonorrhea. As a nurse, what feelings do you anticipate Cindy will experience?	*Nursing Conference* Presentation of a patient situation in which the nurse identifies feelings of a patient who has a diagnosis of a venereal disease.
	Explain your rationale in terms of theories and concepts relevant to the situation	*Criteria* 1. Types of feelings identified 2. Supporting data 3. Completeness of assessment
C2.2 Describes the behavior of elderly people in selected situations.	*Written Assignment* Select two of the following situations and observe for 10 minutes the behavior of an elderly person in terms of: 1. Independent actions 2. Interactions with others 3. Body mannerisms	Observe for 10 minutes the behavior of two elderly hospitalized patients (one, confined to bed, and the other, mobile) in terms of: 1. Independent actions 2. Interactions with others 3. Body mannerisms
	Write up your observations. *Situations* 1. On a bus 2. In a store	Report your observations at a clinical conference.

BEHAVIORAL OBJECTIVE	CLASS EVALUATION	CLINICAL EVALUATION
	3. In church or synagogue	
	4. In a family group	
	5. At a social activity for the elderly	

As with the first illustrations, these two illustrations are included to show the potential for evaluating a particular behavioral objective in both settings of the students' experience—the clinical and the classroom.

PLAN FOR THE EVALUATION OF BEHAVIORAL OBJECTIVES

Teaching, learning, and evaluation all are vibrant, dynamic processes whose characteristics reflect the values, beliefs, and attitudes of participants. The first aspect of the educational process to reflect these individuals is the development of behavioral objectives for the instructional program. The behaviors indicate beliefs about the developmental process of the learner and the nature of the practice by which nurses serve the society. The content indicates the field of knowledge deemed necessary for the behaviors to be actualized.

Once the behaviors and content of the behavioral objectives are identified, planning must provide for operationalizing the behavioral objectives. At this point the character of the teaching-learning process is proclaimed, as the selection of methods and learning experiences is made on the basis of the teacher's concept of the teaching-learning process. The teacher who proposes diverse approaches to operationalizing behavioral objectives is free to individualize the learner's educational experience because options are available.

As is consistent with the concept of unified teaching and learning, the teacher devises evaluation strategies for each behavioral objective. Here, too, diversity is a key factor so that various options are available to the learner. It is to be noted that all of this planning precedes the actual teaching-learning experience. Preplanning of evaluation is particularly important if the relationship between behavioral objectives and the evaluation process is to be maintained.

In too many instances teachers scurry about at evaluation time trying retrospectively to devise some type of examination. The question, "What approaches should I use to evaluate the behavioral objective?" is not the one that is asked. More often questions such as "What material was covered in class?" "Can we ask questions on the readings from the bibliography?" are heard.

When the latter questions control the teacher's development of the evaluation instrument, then the teacher does not perceive the relationship between behavioral objectives and evaluation strategies. If the relationship determines the teacher's evaluation approach, questions as to where the student developed a particular learning would be recognized as irrelevant. The primary concern is the student's mastery of the behavior stated in the objective. Because this is so, evaluation can be developed before the actual course or unit is offered. Preplanning, which also includes alternatives to meet exigencies that may arise in the situation, frees the teacher and the learner alike to devote their energies to the learning process, for both know what will be the focus of the examination during periods of formative and summative evaluation.

EVALUATION AND ACCOUNTABILITY

The importance of maintaining the relationship between behavioral objectives and the evaluation process at all levels of the instructional endeavor, from the individual experience through to the overall program itself, cannot be stressed enough. If behavioral objectives are expressed within a developmental model so that each part of the system contributes to other parts and to the total system itself, then evaluation of behavioral objectives must be developed within the context of the same model. At each point in the system, the integrity of the relationship must be maintained, so that achievement of each behavioral objective can be appraised. The close and contributory interrelationship of behavioral objectives to the total system necessitates that they be evaluated at whatever level in the system they occur. Any evaluation schema that fails to provide for evaluation of each behavioral objective at every level increases risks that incomplete data will be used in making judgments about the practitioner's competency.

Consistency in maintaining the relationship between evaluation strategies and behavioral objectives is not only relevant to the evaluation of the student while in the program, but it is a vital aspect of any program for quality control. When accountability is called for, this does not mean that only the final product is subject to quality control. Each subsystem must meet the demands of accountability, for the total educational endeavor is dependent upon the quality of instruction at each level in the system. A program that states behavioral objectives at each level within a developmental framework and that requires relevant evaluation strategies for each level, is designed to establish accountability for its instructional endeavor.

SUMMARY

A direct relationship exists between the *what* (behavioral objectives) and the *how* (evaluation processes) of an educational endeavor. The relationship is an interdependent one whose character reflects the values and beliefs of participants.

Maintaining the integrity of the relationship is critical if the instructional endeavor is to meet the demands of quality control and if participants are to be held accountable for the quality of the outcome. The declaration of behavioral objectives, their development in a program of studies, and evaluation of their attainment are the processes of education.

Index